# AGE-DEFYING BEAUTY Secrets

## Look and feel younger each and every day

# Diane Irons

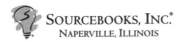 SOURCEBOOKS, INC.®
NAPERVILLE, ILLINOIS

Published by Sourcebooks, Inc.
P.O. Box 4410, Naperville, Illinois 60567-4410
(630) 961-3900
FAX: (630) 961-2168
www.sourcebooks.com

Library of Congress Cataloging-in-Publication Data
Irons, Diane
 Age-defying beauty secrets / by Diane Irons.
   p. cm.
 ISBN 1-4022-0061-7 (alk. paper)
 1. Women—Health and hygiene. 2. Beauty, Personal. 3. Longevity.
4. Youthfulness. I. Title.
RA778 .I7582 2003
613'.04244--dc22
                2003015589

Printed and bound in the United States of America
PX  10  9  8  7  6  5  4  3  2

# DEDICATION

To the two women who shaped my life and formed my character.

My dear mother, who nurtured my sense of self, encouraged my dreams, and gave me her heart and everything else she had. Mom, you sacrificed your life for your children.

My beloved Aunt Stella, who loved me unconditionally and was like a second mother. Your warmth, generous spirit, and compassion will be forever missed.

# ACKNOWLEDGMENTS

I am deeply grateful to the wonderful women who cooperated with me in this book to break the barriers of aging. The surveys, interviews, and discussions were invaluable.

Thanks so much to my friends and colleagues at Sourcebooks for their patience, support, and belief in my words.

To my family and friends, I love you all for understanding when I drop back and "cocoon" myself in the intensity of my projects.

My gratitude goes out to the medical experts who were so generous with their time and knowledge.

I must acknowledge my wonderful readers, who inspire me with their questions and concerns.

# TABLE OF CONTENTS

# Introduction

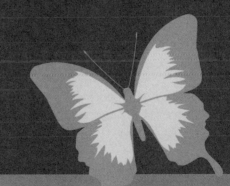

# LET'S LIGHTEN UP

The first-age defying step is to not take aging or yourself so seriously. There are days when we won't look so great. It happens to every one of us eventually. I laugh sometimes when I get out of bed. I could scream, but laughter is a better alternative, especially when I think about legendary beauties who could not handle their changing looks and cocooned themselves in their apartments. Garbo comes to mind, but there have been many others.

Of course, we can't look twenty forever, and we have to accept that life and our looks are changing. We've lived, and it's life affirming to honor our lives by looking into that mirror and saying warmly,

"Hello, old friend." Then promise to pay tribute to that friend by doing a little something that will make it more pleasurable to look again tomorrow.

# GROWING OLD GRACEFULLY

The very word grace means there is something inside of you that will never age, can never grow old. So many women I meet confide, "I know I'm getting old. I see the lines and the sagging. But I don't feel that way. I want to match that feeling inside." In this era, we can make things come together. We have many options.

Some results will come from a bottle, but most will not. Some will take concerted effort, but more important will be a change in attitude. There are other alternatives that can take a little (OK, a lot) of time and money.

It will be your choice how far you want to go, being totally objective and realistic when you look into that mirror and picking back up what you've let slip.

Juggling aging with beauty can seem daunting. My intent is to take the fear out of aging and putting some fun back into your age-defying routines. Each time you do something for yourself, you'll start to feel better, more at ease in your skin. This will create a glow from inside. Trust me, it will be duly noticeable on the outside.

You'll learn what worked at twenty won't succeed at forty. Things you did years ago are now not only not necessary but outdated. Like spending hours on your hair. Sure, it looked great teased and sprayed, but not only will it date you, it's no longer necessary. The good news about the years is that there are new techniques that shave off the beauty routine minutes. Soft and natural is the way to go so you can prevent looking like a caricature of your former self. You cannot hairspray the years away. It's time to move out of the time warp.

# MAKE PEACE WITH YOUR AGE

You'll never be eighteen again, and all things should and must pass. Time heals and time teaches. We can't have exactly what we think we want: that young, perky body to go along with our years of wisdom.

When should age defying start? Early. As soon as possible. It starts with good habits. Some we never had, but it's never too late to start—simple habits like wearing sunscreen, eating the right foods, and giving up or at the very least moderating alcohol and smoking.

When does it end? It's doesn't. Giving up on your looks is akin to giving up on life. As long as you can gaze into a mirror, as often as you interact with anything or anyone, you owe it to yourself to do something.

It's respectful to your spirit, and it's a sign of respect to others.

# Chapter 1

# AGE-DEFYING ATTITUDE

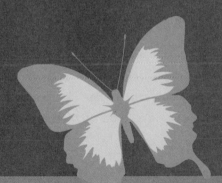

# HOW WILL YOU AGE?

No matter what your age, twenty-five or fifty-five, aging is something that weighs on a woman's mind.

We are an age-driven, youth-obsessed culture. We look at pictures in magazines that have been airbrushed or computer stretched and believe that since we cannot live up to those standards, why even bother? Look, it's their livelihood to look that good and that young. But what about the rest of us? We don't have the money, the time, or the single-visioned reality to want to live that way. It would be pretty boring to have to live like that, anyway. But there is something that we all have—a mindset. If we can change our attitudes and remake the rules for aging, we can defy age right down the line.

Ironically, a woman in her twenties is the most insecure about her looks. This is because she is more likely to try to believe that she can obtain perfection. If she diets, it's not for health reasons, it's for her weight. As we age, it becomes more about health, and that's the way it should be.

Women today are defying age more than ever because we have more freedom to do it. We have the ability to live our lives the way we want. We've broken out of the box. We have more options. We can marry or not, we can go to school when we want, we can delay child-bearing and control the number of children we have. We can have careers or stay at home.

We shouldn't feel trapped. Aging well is now a choice. Successful age defying is the result of making an effort. Just because you've reached a certain age, you still want to look and feel as good as you possibly can for as long as you can.

## YOU AND YOUR MOTHER

Your mother is a good indicator of how you will age. However, if you look more like your father, you might age this way. For instance, if your

2

father has dark spots on his skin, you should avoid the sun.

## YOUR FACE **STRUCTURE**

The rule is the fuller your face, the more it will sag.

You'll first notice eyebrows drooping, causing you to look tired and people to ask you if you're tired when you're not. The jawline will begin to sag. These areas are the first to aggressively treat.

## YOU CAN **SLOW DOWN** YOUR CLOCK

There are age-defying techniques that do make the difference. From what you eat to how you think, it all adds up.

## WHAT'S YOUR **OUTLOOK**?

Would you say that you're "young at heart"? If you let your chronological age affect how you conduct your life or your attitude toward your looks, you're going to have to change.

## TRY **SOMETHING NEW**

It doesn't have to be a new haircut. It could be a new and healthy food or exercise, a new store to shop, or even a new beauty procedure. If you need to slowly adjust your attitude, that's a start. It's a good beginning.

## WATCH YOUR **LANGUAGE**

Never say, "When I was young." The only correct term is, "When I was younger."

You need to hold yourself in the same esteem as you hold others.

## MAKE IT **PLAY**

When it's fun, it makes you immediately younger. A playful attitude is a beauty treatment on its own.

## IT'S A **DAILY** DECISION

What you do each day can take away your looks or add to them.

## GET ENOUGH **SLEEP**

It will keep your metabolism revved up. Plus, not getting enough of it will zap your energy so that you'll act like an old grandma.

## WATCH YOUR **DRINKING**

There's a lot of controversy about how much is too much. The general consensus is that a glass of wine a day may actually be beneficial to your health. Very heavy drinking can cause broken blood vessels, dry patches, and an unattractive gray pallor.

## **EAT** SOMETHING

Nutrition plays such an important part in how you look. There are antioxidants from fruits and vegetables that no cream can provide.

## WATER, THE **FREE**, **READY-TO-GO** BEAUTY TREATMENT

Drinking water keeps skin hydrated and glowing. It's the number-one way to feel younger and healthier.

## **SMOKING**: A BEAUTY AND HEALTH RISK

You already know that cigarettes are linked to cancer, but smoking also decreases blood flow to your skin and causes wrinkles and yellowing.

## fountain of youth

**Did you know that chewing gum can give you wrinkles? Just like smoking, the repetitive motion creates lines and wrinkles around the mouth.**

## CALM DOWN

Anger causes frown lines. When you're angry, you speed up your heart rate, raising your blood pressure. Take deep breaths when you're stuck in line, in traffic, or otherwise annoyed.

But don't keep it in. There's nothing like standing up for what you believe in to get the blood flowing.

## STRESS

Just look at our presidents as they enter office and then again as they leave office. Enough said.

## THINK ABOUT SOMETHING **PLEASANT**

Take a little mind excursion. But don't keep your frustrations inside your body. It's not healthy.

## **LAUGH** A LOT

Laughing reduces stress and physical tension. Don't catastrophize. You don't need to do this anymore. You need to reevaluate what is important and what isn't.

Did you mess up? At least you gave it a shot.

Your plans fell through…so make others!

# AGE-DEFYING RULES

❖ There can never be too much sunscreen.
❖ Don't bother using a moisturizer if it doesn't have antioxidants.
❖ You can't stop time, but you can definitely slow it down.

## **BREATHE** DEEPLY

Scientists are finding that meditation helps keep wrinkles away and the body healthy.

## KEEP **HANGING IN**

Don't give up and go into a deep depression the first time some kid calls you "ma'am." Remember when you saw someone who had let herself go, and you wondered why? "Why" sounds more reasonable than "why not?"

## ALWAYS CHOOSE **COMFORT**

You deserve it after all those years of lying down on your bed trying to zip up your jeans.

But there's a big difference between comfort and sloppiness.

## GIVE YOURSELF **LITTLE PLEASURES**

Schedule breaks for yourself. Don't try to keep going until you drop.

## CREATE A **REGIMEN**

Your body will react positively to having a regular schedule. Not only will it make your lifestyle simpler and more enjoyable, it will allow you to get more into your day.

Make sure that your schedule is reasonable and fits your lifestyle. Don't create a schedule that you are forced to adapt to.

## YES, YOU CAN **TEACH AN OLD DOG**

You can learn good habits that will help turn back the clock.

## SAVE PRECIOUS **TIME**

❖ Use products that perform more than one task.
❖ Rely on products that are easy to use, like a blush that gently lights up your skin, lipstick that doesn't need a magnifying mirror, and moisturizer with sunscreen added.

## YOU GOTTA HAVE **FRIENDS**

Having women and female relatives to talk to doesn't just keep you from feeling lonely, it has been scientifically documented to rev up the immune system, according to research from the University of Michigan. Women supporting one another can add to esteem, helping you feel more worthy and competent. The research indicates that you don't need a lot of friends, just reliable ones. An interesting side note to the research is that having too many friends is not necessarily healthy because women tend to be caretakers in relationships. Friendships can be demanding.

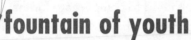

## fountain of youth

**Having a dog as a friend can lower blood pressure. Romantic love is not the only kind of love to nurture.**

## LOVING YOURSELF ALSO BOOSTS YOUR HEALTH

## MOVE

We wish there was an anti-aging pill, but there is something that's close. It's exercise. Studies have shown that exercise keeps skin firm and strengthens the heart, lungs, bones, and muscles. It stimulates the production of antioxidants in the body as well as boosting the immune system.

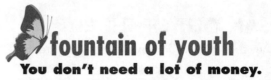

## fountain of youth

**You don't need a lot of money.**
**The less you have, the easier it is to manage.**

> "WE ARE ALWAYS THE SAME AGE INSIDE."
>
> —Gertrude Stein

## BREAK SOME RULES

There are no rules anymore when it comes to looking great. If you're in need of age defying, trying something as small as adding some new colors or shimmer on top of what is your own. For instance, if you just love that red lipstick you've worn since you were sixteen, perhaps you can bring it up to date with a gloss.

7

## BREAK OUT OF THE RUT

You may think that your look is absolutely great, but change something for a day.

You can always go back if it doesn't improve things. Then go out and see if anyone notices.

## PAY ATTENTION

Your body and mind will tell you what you need, when it's time to change, when it's time to leave, when you need a surge of energy, and when you need to cut back.

## KNOW YOURSELF

Know what looks good on you and what doesn't.

## BE REASONABLE

If the skin on your arms is hanging down, don't wear sleeveless shirts until you can do something about them. Why bring yourself down? On the other hand, if your legs are still great, keep on wearing those short skirts. Again, be reasonable and consider short to be just above the knee.

## IT'S ALL ABOUT SELF PRESERVATION

Become more interested in skin care. Learn all you can about the changes in your body.

For instance, your oil glands are starting to give out. You need to compensate for that.

Realize that skin photosensitizes on the neck and can be damaged as a result of the usual method of applying fragrance on the side of the neck. Start applying fragrance to other areas.

## DON'T FADE INTO THE WOODWORK

Some women think that as they age, they should become invisible. So they stay safe.

Then they hate it. Look, if you don't want to bring attention to your crow's feet, emphasize your eyebrows.

## GLAMOUR IS AGELESS

With just the right amount of fragrance and jewelry, a pair of heels, and an attitude sprinkled with a large dose of confidence, glamour comes about. Too much of anything is just the opposite.

## LEARN TO **COMPENSATE**

You can reduce your risk of middle-age spread by reducing your food intake or upping your activity level.

Rebuild your muscle mass with strength training. Muscle is lost with age.

Get more fiber into your diet to make up for your digestive system slowing down.

> "Nature gives you the face you have at twenty; it is up to you to merit the face you have at fifty."
>
> —Coco Chanel

# GENERAL GUIDELINES

## MAINTAIN A **HEALTHY WEIGHT**

Gaining a few extra pounds as we age shouldn't be cause for alarm, but it is a warning sign. Once you gain more than twenty pounds in adulthood, physicians warn that you're at an increased risk of diabetes, hypertension, and heart disease.

## START **LIFTING WEIGHTS**

Starting around age forty, women lose about a half a pound of muscle each year because of slowed metabolism, gaining roughly the same amount of fat. However, with strength training, age-related changes can be kept under control.

## GET ENOUGH **CALCIUM**

Calcium affects most major organs and plays an important role in controlling blood pressure, preserving bones, and preventing some cancers. The nutrition research center at Tufts University in Medford, Massachusetts states that calcium is best taken from food, but if that's not possible, supplements are second best.

## WHO NEEDS **STRESS**?

No, I'm not being unrealistic about our chaotic world, but we've really become a culture trained to think of aging as loss. What about all that you've gained and what you've learned?

## WHAT'S **GOING ON**?

Most confusing and aggravating is getting strange things like acne as we age. Strange things like this happen because aging is not a straightforward process. It's a constant up and down and back and forth.

So even though you've never had problems with your skin, you might have problems now because nature is beginning to catch up with you and your hormones are acting up.

## MAKE **SMALL** CHANGES

It will look better to enhance your features rather than try to change them at your age.

How great you look isn't all about hair and makeup. The way you carry yourself is just as important. The way you think about yourself is key. The way you present yourself for the world is what makes all the difference.

## AGING **WELL** COMES FROM DEEP **WITHIN**

So what if you're not a size eight or your thighs have dimples? Concentrate on what's great about your body. You may have great shoulders. Bring the eye there.

The great thing about aging well is that you don't have to prove anything to anybody but yourself.

Don't try to look too matchy matchy. We are no longer at the age (thank goodness) where we want to look like we're trying too hard. It can look pathetic, quite frankly.

## KEEP **UPDATING**

❖ With each decade comes the need to reassess everything.

❖ You need to try new things.

❖ You need to go out and find out what is new in the world.

# GET OUT OF THAT RUT

❖ Check to see if you're wearing the same colors or variations on a theme of fashion. Skin tone changes over the years and even seasonally. You need to keep revamping.

❖ Don't panic if more than one of your favorite products has been discontinued. There's a reason for discontinuing a product. Textures change, color themes come and go, and new concepts make products better and better. If it's gone, it's gone for a good reason.

❖ Mix up your cosmetics colors. Lighten up in the summer, darken down in the winter. Wearing pink or gloss is not only wrong, it's not flattering during some seasons.

❖ Don't panic if you find yourself starting to gain weight. Just up your exercise and keep flexible. You don't have to become an acrobat; however, you have to keep moving. Walking is a great general conditioning exercise, and you don't need any money or equipment to walk.

## STAND UP **STRAIGHT**

Posture says it all. The way we carry ourselves can immediately make us appear more attractive and younger. You could have the most expensive, exquisite outfit, the most extensive surgery, and the most artfully applied makeup, but if you

11

don't have the body or carriage to carry it on, they're not going to do a thing for you.

## DON'T BE AFRAID

If we can start looking at aging as a transformation, then we can stop being afraid of it.

## YOU KNOW YOUR STYLE

The secret to age-defying aging is to keep your style intact. You know what you're comfortable in, and it should take precedence over any trend.

## STAY FULLY ALIVE

Don't ever give up on yourself. Just because your beauty changes doesn't mean it stops being beautiful.

## AGE IS ONLY A NUMBER

It has nothing to do with how you look and it has everything to do with how well you've lived your life.

## KEEP YOUR BALANCE

Stay healthy by picking the right workout video and the healthy foods that you like to eat.

If you do the things that you like to do and you eat the things that you like, then you're aging with balance and you will keep doing it for life.

# STAY CONNECTED!

The goal is to develop yourself through your relationships. Each relationship should nurture you and support you as you reach your goals.

## LET YOUR SPIRIT GUIDE YOU

You have only so much control in this world. Focus on being happy with what you have.

## GET SOMETHING DONE

❖ Even a small accomplishment a day makes you feel good.

❖ Focus until you finish.

❖ Create goals that are truly achievable.

## THE **FOCUS** IS YOU

Do what comes naturally.

Make the most of what you were given, not what you wish you were given.

## RELAX

You have to know what you can and can't control.

## **GO BACK** IN TIME

❖ Rent a convertible if you don't have one and put on those old tunes. You'll instantly feel "that" age, and go back to "that" summer of love.

❖ Pick a look out of a magazine, put it up on your mirror, and try to copy it.

❖ Pick something modern, fun, and achievable.

## GET AN **OBJECTIVE** OPINION

Find a friend, grab a bottle of wine, and do each other's makeup. Be honest with each other, and take pictures to mark the event.

## fountain of youth

**Do your best every day. Look your best every day.**

**Yes, I know it's not easy, but you'll sleep better at night knowing you've done your best.**

## KEEP YOUR **EYES OPEN**

Stay excited by new things that come along. Stay up to date on fashion trends and new age-defying techniques. It will keep your eye young.

## RAISE YOUR **BROWS/** RAISE YOUR **ATTITUDE**

It forces the corners of your eyes up, and that little smile booster will go right inside to the core of you. Studies have linked smiling to chemical changes that relax the body and can even lift mood.

## **LIVE YOUNGER** WITH A FEW ALTERATIONS

Life should be fun, not too safe and not too risky.

## AGE IS **JUST A NUMBER**

With so many external beauty treatments that address aging, attitude is the only one that really matters. Your mood will be better, people will notice and respect you, and you'll have a better day. And, most important, the world will seem a little warmer.

# Chapter 2

# AGE-DEFYING SKIN

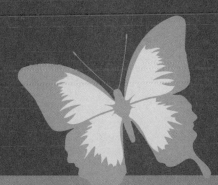

# SKIN CHANGES

Remember that smooth, flawless skin you used to take for granted? It's not there anymore, is it? In the battle to defy age, caring for your skin is the first line of defense.

Of course, everything changes. It's natural, right? Well, it doesn't have to be that way.

There are a lot of conscious decisions that will help to minimize and even delay aging of the skin.

## WHAT'S **HAPPENING**?

Your skin has lost pigment through the years. The surface has roughened. The immune cells you were born with have been lessened (by as much as 50 percent!). Your glow is gone. Less oxygen is being carried to the surface of the skin.

## **MEN'S** SKIN/ **WOMEN'S** SKIN

Although women live an average of eight years longer than men, our skin looks older.

That's because men's skin is thicker and they have those facial follicles that hold their skin in place.

Most men don't stand in front of the mirror checking out every crinkle, sag, and scar.

That's because they don't have them as soon as we do.

## YOUR **COLLAGEN** IS SLOWING DOWN

Sun damage and the whole aging process cause women to lose collagen, the substance that keeps our skin together. The collagen fibers twist and mat so that the skin begins to line, sag, and wrinkle. Also, your skin is losing the ability to hold water, causing it to become drier.

Oil production also diminishes.

## **HORMONAL** CHANGES

When women are in their twenties, they have more female hormones (estrogens) than male hormones (androgens). As women age, the ratio starts to change and estrogen production slows down. Estrogen keeps skin soft and elastic. This not only causes skin wrinkling but other skin conditions such as rosacea and acne.

So all these changes, depressing as they seem, are nature's less-than-subtle way of reminding us of our age. We can defy these gentle nudges. It's never too early, and there is no such thing as too late.

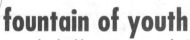# fountain of youth

**Rosacea looks like an acne rash. It can also resemble a persistent flush. Benzoyl peroxide is an inexpensive and effective treatment.**

## **EASY** DOES IT

Too much washing is not only unnecessary, it can aggravate and irritate fragile, aging skin. Your skin is a living organ, and your body's largest. It's the first reminder of your lifestyle, your personal choices, and self care. It's not a floor to scrub.

Every night, take about a teaspoon of cold cream or other mild cleanser, apply it to a coarse cloth, and remove all makeup. Massage cream into the skin of the face and neck, starting at the neck, using an upward motion from the center to the sides. Rinse thoroughly with warm water. Then rinse the cloth, dip it into a small amount of witch hazel, and dab gently on skin. This will remove any residue and excess without stripping oils.

Finish by splashing cool water to close pores and stimulate circulation. Allow skin to air dry just a bit before applying moisturizer. Moisturizer not only helps skin retain moisture, it also protects it from the environment.

## MORNING ROUTINE

Your nighttime moisturizer should still be doing its work and your face should be slightly moist with a few oils. The worst thing you put on your face is soap. But you do need to wake yourself up and reactivate your moisturizer as well as get rid of any extra oil accumulation.

That's right. A positive benefit of age defying is that some things get easier. A splash of cool water on your face, and you're ready to go.

# SKIN COMMANDO

In the quest to fight aging, the skin is the place to start. You'll notice almost immediate results, which will motivate you to begin other anti-aging tactics.

Is it time to start fighting back? Although it's important to maintain a lifestyle of quality skin care, look for these obvious signs of aging to see if you need to become more aggressive.

❖ You pull at the skin on the top of your hand and it takes more than a second or two to spring back.

❖ You get a lot of face creasing when you sleep, and it lasts longer than it used to.

❖ Your skin feels tight.

❖ You are seeing flaking on areas of skin.

❖ You look constantly fatigued.

❖ It's time to switch from maintenance products to treatment options.

## CELL RENEWAL

Since your skin is starting to slow down, you need to accelerate the process by using products containing alpha hydroxy acids. Try to find products that contain anti-inflammatory ingredients like allantoin or panthenol. Renewing the cells, turning over dead skin, makes skin more vibrant. If your skin has become dull, you need to add this skin treatment.

## TEXTURE

You're also producing less sebum, so moisturizers are vital. Look for antioxidant additives, which will also help fight damage from free radicals.

# COMMON SENSE

## WATCH WHAT YOU **PUT ON** YOUR FACE

That means no telephones on the chin, hands cupping the face, fingers picking at pimples, or anything that can stretch your skin or cause additional wrinkling.

## WATCH **WHERE YOU PUT** YOUR FACE

Sleeping with your face pressed against a pillow can cause wrinkling in the same way repeating facial expressions can. Although you certainly don't want to stop laughing to eliminate laugh lines, you can prevent sleep wrinkling.

❖ Learn to sleep on your back. It's uncomfortable at first, but easy to learn.

❖ Exchange your current pillowcase for a satin one. Its finish will cause your face to slip and slide and prevent creasing.

❖ Use a neck roll in addition to your pillow to extend your neck and take the pressure off your face.

❖ Choose a smaller pillow. Try to keep the size down so there's less surface to damage skin. Plus, a smaller pillow allows your face to control the pillow rather than the pillow taking over your face.

# WRINKLE MANAGEMENT

Your habits can contribute greatly to aging skin. Unconscious bad behaviors that have developed over the years can be conquered.

Throughout the day, there are ways to combat wrinkling that just require a little conscious effort. In very little time, the new habit takes over and becomes automatic.

Try not to turn down the corners of your mouth when you're deep in thought, reading a book, at your computer, etc. Put a mirror near you to check yourself.

Check yourself to make sure that you're not squinting while reading or at the computer.

If you are, talk to your optometrist to make sure that it's not a vision problem.

## DON'T RUB!

Excessive eye rubbing is not only an unattractive habit, it can cause the skin around the eye to become loose and saggy.

### fountain of youth

**Don't go out in the sunlight without sunglasses.** You don't need to encourage more lines from squinting.

## USE YOUR HANDS

If you have very sensitive skin, use your hands to cleanse rather than a coarse washcloth.

Your fingers can fit nicely into the crevices of your nose and push cleanser into the eye area with just enough pressure.

## HAPPY HANDS

Rub cold sore medicine like Herpecin L on your hands when they're feeling dry to heal them quickly. Herpecin contains zinc oxide, which also helps with diaper rash.

# KNOW YOUR INGREDIENTS

Products claim to do all sorts of things to prevent and reverse aging, but you need to read the ingredient labels to be sure that they're doing what they're supposed to do.

❖ **Alpha hydroxy acids** loosen dead cells from skin's surface.

❖ **Antioxidants** fight free radicals that accelerate aging.

❖ **Anti-inflammatories** reduce puffiness.

❖ **Emollients** form a protective film to trap moisture.

❖ **Exfoliants** remove dead skin cells and debris.

❖ **Fatty acids** protect the skin barrier.

❖ **Humectants** attract moisture from the atmosphere and bond it to the skin.

❖ **Hyaluronic acid** helps skin maintain proper moisture levels.

❖ **Vitamins** added to products provide great benefits.

❖ **Vitamin A** improves skin elasticity, promotes a more even texture, and promotes new cell growth.

❖ **Vitamin C** enhances collagen production for firmer skin.

❖ **Vitamin E** adds moisture and repairs tissue.

Here's a good way to choose a MOISTURIZER for AGING SKIN: dab a little on a tissue. If it leaves an OILY STAIN, it's a good candidate because it will have sufficient oil to protect skin.

# HOME REMEDIES

Age defying can be done very effectively and inexpensively at home with these age-defying recipes that are cheap and a cinch to make!

## ASPIRIN EXFOLIATORS

Mash three aspirin and let dissolve in a half teaspoon of lemon juice and half teaspoon water.

Gently massage on face and let set for two to three minutes.

Rinse. You'll immediately see brighter skin, plus this mask helps rid skin of discoloration.

## SUPER SKIN FIRMER

Combine one quarter cup plain yogurt with two teaspoons brewer's yeast.

Add a teaspoon of wine vinegar.

Spread over face and neck.

Allow to set for fifteen minutes and then rinse with apple cider vinegar and water (equal amounts).

## BRIGHTENING MASK

Add one packet unflavored gelatin to one half cup apple juice.

Heat in the microwave for about thirty seconds. Refrigerate until set.

Spread over face and allow to dry.

Rinse with tepid water.

## CIRCULATION-STIMULATING MASK

Combine a teaspoon of cornstarch with about six mashed grapes.

Pat over face and let set for about fifteen minutes.

Rinse first with warm water, then cool water.

## WRINKLE-SOFTENING MASK

Mash half a cucumber and apply to clean, dry skin.

Leave on at least fifteen minutes before rinsing with cool water.

## AT-HOME **PEEL**

This inexpensive at-home acid peel is so easy!

Simply soak a cotton ball in apple cider vinegar and apply over face, avoiding eyes.

It will sting slightly, so keep eyes closed. Keep on at least thirty minutes.

This is a great mask for treating old acne scars.

# AGE-DEFYING LIPS

Your lips are so important because the skin there is so fragile. Plus, lips don't have oil glands, so they require extra care.

## STOP LICKING YOUR LIPS!

It seems when you are licking your lips that you are hydrating them, but the opposite is true. The saliva you added quickly evaporates and destroys any moisture or protection that was originally there. So your lips end up even drier. It can become an endless cycle.

## BRUSH YOUR **TEETH/** BRUSH YOUR **LIPS**

Exfoliate your lips each night before applying moisturizer. After brushing your teeth, gently brush your lips. Then apply eye moisturizer or lip balm. A coarse washcloth works in the morning to exfoliate lips.

## fountain of youth

**To make your lip balm even more effective, heat it for a couple of seconds in the microwave, or spot heat it with your hair dryer.**

## AGE-DEFYING **HANDS**

Your hands are fragile due to the very thin skin on them. They can give away your age years before your face does. The best way to keep your hands protected is to always apply sunscreen with an SPF of at least 30. Look for a sunscreen that has emollients or add a vitamin E capsule to it upon application.

## AGE-DEFYING **NECK**

Always apply moisturizer to the neck as well as the face. If your neck is heavily lined, apply eye concentrate.

> **Because the skin of the neck is so sensitive, AVOID EXFOLIATING SCRUBS in this area.**

## CLEAVAGE

The chest area is prone to sagging and freckles, and this is a sure sign of aging.

It is too often neglected because it is under cover. And yet, it is one of the most sensuous areas of your body!

Now, more than ever, your cleavage is begging for exfoliation, moisturizing, and, of course, sun protection.

Apply 2 percent hydroquinone to age spots, avoiding any moles or other suspicious spots. They should be checked out by your health care provider.

**Use a SCRUBBING BRUSH in your shower as well as an EXFOLIANT for the chest area.**

**You need to PROTECT THIS AREA even in cold weather.**

**Don't forget the MOISTURIZER year round.**

# PROGRESSIVE PROBLEMS

## LARGE PORES

Pores become larger with age because skin tissue breaks down as it ages. This is more noticeable around pores. Although you can't shrink them, you can shrink their appearance, and you can slow skin degeneration down.

❖ Use a mild astringent to temporarily tighten pores.
❖ Avoid the sun and concentrate sunscreen on the enlarged pores.
❖ Drink plenty of water for skin hydration and blood flow.
❖ Limit caffeine.

## CELLULITE

It progresses as we age and skin loses elasticity. Massage and caffeinated products work best.

## AGE SPOTS

Lighten them with lemon juice.

Fade them away with hydroquinone. You can purchase 2 percent strength without a prescription.

## DRYING AND CRACKING

❖ Use a humidifier or place a pan of water on the radiator in your bedroom.
❖ Take short showers and baths, especially during winter.
❖ Keep the temperature of the water warm, not hot.
❖ Add bath oils.

If you are taking a **DIURETIC**, it may be increasing the dryness of your skin. Diuretics **DRY THE SKIN** internally.

# TOPICAL TREATMENTS

## FACIALS

Whether you do it yourself or have it done professionally, if you're over thirty, a facial is beneficial.

A good facial:

- ❖ Exfoliates to allow younger cells to surface
- ❖ Unclogs pores to allow treatments to penetrate.
- ❖ Hydrates skin.

Don't have a facial is your skin is sun- or windburned.

A facial should not cause any post-treatment breakouts.

## EYE CREAMS

Look for a cream specially formulated for this area. Always choose the least-fragrant eye cream available. This delicate area can be easily irritated.

Added ingredients to look for: retinol, vitamin C.

To make eye treatments feel more soothing, store them in the refrigerator.

## MASSAGE

Sagging and puffiness can be improved through massage. Massage can also help another aging problem: circulation. Improving circulation will eliminate toxins and greatly improve skin tone. Improving skin tone aids firming.

1. Place the fingertips of each hand below the bottom lashes of each eye. Very slowly, push the skin of your lower lids upward, being careful not to wrinkle your forehead as you do. Push both lids as high as you can. Relax a moment and then repeat five times more.

2. Place three fingers of your left hand very gently on the right side of your face from the corner of your right nostril down to the corner of your mouth. Then gently press your right thumb on the outside corner of your right eye and the remaining fingers of your right hand on the area just above and between your eyebrows. Wink your right eye as you lift the right side of your mouth. Wink and lift at the same time. Do this ten times and then repeat on the left side of your face.

# STRANGE BUT TRUE

## VAGINAL CREAMS?

Some women will try anything! And buy anything. I mean, they're turning to vaginal creams to treat facial wrinkles. The rationale is that since the cream is helpful in alleviating vaginal dryness, irritation, and itching among menopausal women by stimulating collagen formation in the vagina, it could also stimulate collagen formation in facial skin.

# SUPPLEMENTS

## DMAE
Naturally found in high levels in fish, it smoothes out dimpling and firms skin.

## VITAMIN C ESTER
Increases the production of collagen, which helps thicken skin.

## ALPHA LIPOIC ACID
Treats fine lines and wrinkles, enlarged pores, and puffiness.

## GINSENG
Boosts circulation and oxygenation.

# PROBLEMS AND SOLUTIONS

## MENOPAUSE
Skin can become extremely dry and rough during menopause.

Make sure you're drinking enough water to compensate for what's happening inside your body.

Add flaxseed oil to your daily diet (two tablespoons is the recommended dosage).

Install a chlorine filter in your showerhead. Chlorine can be extremely drying.

Add fatty fish to your diet three or four times a week.

# Chapter 3

# AGE-DEFYING BODIES

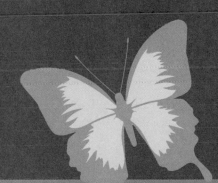

# SIGNS OF AGING

What's happening here? It seems like everything is starting to drop on our bodies. And it's happening fast!

Bone mass starts to decline in the mid to late thirties. Women can lose as much as 1 percent of their total bone mass each year until menopause.

If you don't exercise on a regular basis, you can lose up to 30 percent of your muscle weight by the time you reach seventy. Losing muscle results in the reduction of metabolism, making it harder for your body to burn calories.

## ELASTICITY

Skin gradually starts to lose elasticity, and that means skin starts to wrinkle.

Skin will become drier as less sebum is produced.

## CELL RENEWAL

The rate of cell renewal slows down, which causes skin to look duller.

Skin becomes thinner and looks looser.

## FAT STORAGE

Fat is stored as we age because our bodies need less food and we tend to be less active than ever before.

## WHAT CAN BE CHANGED?

First, let me tell you what can't be changed.

You can't change your body type. And you can't change where your fat collects.

You can't regain bone loss.

If you tend to gain weight in your stomach, that's the first place it will go and the last place it will leave.

❖ You can change your fat level. This can make a major difference in your shape.
❖ You can change the amount of fat that you store through diet and exercise.

❖ You can change your muscle tone. It will create a sleeker, firmer shape.

# BODY BATTLES

You can keep your body from aging faster than it needs to, and you can do it without a personal trainer or a visit to a chi-chi spa.

## VISUALIZATION

Imagine what the results of eating better, getting enough exercise, and generally taking care of your body will feel like. Imagine how happy you'll be and how much more energy you'll have. Think about the sense of well-being and the sense of control.

Take yourself on this journey of the mind and it will make it more achievable.

## DON'T GET STUCK ON A SCALE

A scale is only one way to gauge your health and physicality. Keep a tape measure in the bathroom to keep track of your waist measurement, which increases with age. Plus, a scale can't recognize the seven glasses of water that you've had in the last two hours.

You can go crazy living by the scale.

## LISTEN TO YOUR BODY

Everyone has bad days, but a big change in your energy level is not to be ignored.

Pay attention to these and other changes and report them to your doctor if they continue.

## KEEP MOVING

Take a walk every day, take the stairs instead of the elevator, do some stretches to keep your body energized.

## BE REALISTIC

You probably will not be able to bounce a quarter off your butt again, and you'll waste too much of your precious time trying to get there. There comes a time in your life when you need to know that your body is not meant to go

31

below a certain weight to be healthy and to have the necessary energy to keep up your daily activities.

## SLOW DOWN

You need to rest; otherwise, your body becomes overstimulated. This is a big body aging factor. Even if it's just five minutes, go outside and breathe deeply. Close your eyes for ten minutes. Little breaks like these will lower your heart rate and stress hormone levels.

# AGE-DEFYING EXERCISES

## ARM TONING

Kimono arms, flag wavers, here's an exercise to stop them.

Stand with feet shoulder width apart and knees slightly relaxed. Bend arms and hold fists in front of your face, facing inward. Punch your right fist across to an imaginary opponent's left shoulder. Repeat twenty-five times, and then repeat in the same way with your left fist to the opponent's right shoulder.

## BACK TONER

This can be done while you're driving, and it's a great one to get rid of bra bulges.

Press your shoulder blades into the back of your seat while you correct your posture.

Hold for thirty seconds. Repeat several times during the day.

## UPPER BODY STRENGTHENING

This exercise is important for good posture—which starts to go downhill as we age—and for total body alignment.

Hold a five-pound weight in each hand, slightly in front of your thighs with your palms facing inward. Relax your shoulders and bend your elbows as you raise the weight to your chest. Be sure to keep your hands close to your body.

Slowly lower and repeat ten times.

## WAIST TRIMMER

Sitting on a chair, place your feet flat on the floor, shoulder width part.

Inhale as you lift your right arm to the ceiling, then exhale as you bend to the left until your upper body is parallel to the floor.

Inhale as you return to your original position.

Repeat with the left arm.

Try to work up to ten times a day.

## FANNY FIRMER

Using the wall for support makes this exercise kinder to your knees and forces your glutes to get the benefits.

Lean against a wall and slide down until hips are level with knees and knees are directly over ankles.

Hold for thirty seconds.

Slide back to start position and repeat four more times.

## BUST LIFTER

This exercise works on the pectoral muscles and creates the same resistance as a push up.

Stand holding a tennis ball in front of you. Place your hands on the sides of the ball and press it as hard as you can (as if you are trying to pop it).

Hold each squeeze as long as you can (at least thirty seconds).

Repeat up to ten times.

## INNER THIGH TONER

I love this exercise because you can do it when you're talking on the phone or watching your favorite show.

Stand with your right hand against a wall to balance.

Lift your left leg out to the side as far as you can without leaning your body to the right.

Hold your leg up for at least thirty seconds.

Repeat with your left hand/right leg.

Do this five times.

This exercise also helps with balance and posture.

## **TUMMY** TUCK

Here's another exercise that can be done any-where and any time.

Contract the muscles of your stomach and hold for thirty seconds. Repeat five times.

## GARDENING

The University of Arkansas reported results of a study of women over fifty.

Those with the highest bone density were those who worked out with weights or did yard work. Gardening beat out swimming and walk-ing in fighting osteoporosis.

## EXERCISE SMARTER

It's easy to exercise if you incorporate it into your daily life. As you age, you'll need to walk farther as your metabolism slows down. Introduce strength training for thirty minutes each week. Vary your strides when you walk. Take a different route. Walk with weights. Check with your doctor to see if you can handle a few sprints in your walk.

To lose a pound of fat in a week, you must CONSUME 500 FEWER calories or BURN 500 calories daily MORE than necessary to maintain your current weight.

## STAND UP STRAIGHTER

Not only does good posture make you look slimmer and taller, but when the spine is out of balance, the rest of the body compensates. Daily stresses and tensions can wear you down. Muscles tighten up and shorten, become over-stretched and weak.

When your spine is out of alignment, your muscles have to work twice as hard to stabilize the body, and your entire body is more prone to pain and injury.

People with poor posture are using energy just to stand up!

# FAT BURNING

There are secrets to burning fat that come in the form of supplements. Check with your physician before adding these or any supplementation to your diet. Research has found that these supplements not only pump up your energy, they stimulate your body to burn fat and build lean muscle tissue.

## COENZYME Q10

This supplement is useful for obesity, coronary heart disease, lack of energy, and high cholesterol levels. Studies have found that supplementation with up to 150 milligrams of Q10 helps with keeping metabolism energized.

## CONJUGATED LINOLEIC ACID

Commonly known as CLA, this is a fatty acid that occurs naturally in dairy products and red meat. It helps cells convert protein, fat, and carbohydrates into energy. The studies that have been done were on 4.2 grams daily. The results are that food is burned more efficiently, burning body fat as well. Research indicates that results are seen within two weeks.

## CHROMIUM

Scientific studies have discovered that people who lack chromium in their bodies carry extra weight. The supplements chromium picolinate and chromium polynicotate are available at drugstores and health food stores. Some users have reported that chromium is helpful in cutting cravings for sweets. The recommended daily dosage is 400 micrograms.

## L-CARNITINE

This supplement accelerates the benefits of chromium. L-Carnitine is an amino acid that shuttles fat into the cells' energy. The recommendation is for 1,500 milligrams of L-Carnitine in combination with chromium.

## WHEY PROTEIN

This byproduct of milk and yogurt reportedly increases the production of lean muscle by 50 percent and increases fat burning. Whey protein is sold as a powder that is mixed into shakes. You can find whey protein in health food stores.

# AGE-DEFYING BODY TRICKS

## BARING ARMS

Lean over a chair and hold a five pound weight at your side. Lay your free hand flat on the chair. Bring weight up behind you slowly and hold to the count of five. Repeat ten times and then switch sides.

Before wearing anything sleeveless, mix a few drops of lemon juice and olive oil with enough sea salt to make a coarse paste. Massage briskly over arms and then rinse.

## A LEG UP

Run up and down a flight of stairs five or six times. This is a great way to keep your legs toned without any equipment, and it's an effective form of cardio.

## FAT-FIGHTING MASSAGE

While in the shower, starting at the knees, knead skin with your knuckles in an upward motion to break up the fat deposits.

## LEG SLIMMING ILLUSION

Mix a tablespoon of baby oil with a few drops of foundation and apply to legs.

# Chapter 4

# AGE-DEFYING CELEBRITIES

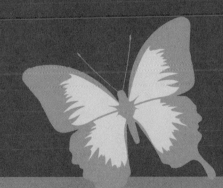

No matter what their age, celebrities make it their job to look as young and slim as possible. They have some unique tips, and some you've probably heard before, but it's always helpful to see how they struggle with our very same issues.

### Christina Applegate

Here is a successful actress who believes in consolidation as her key for looking great on the run. She carries multitask items, such as lipstick that doubles as blush.

### Catherine Dent

Lip balm is her secret weapon. She keeps it on her bedside at night and puts it on her lips and cuticles to soften.

### Rebecca Romijn-Stamos

A bronzing stick is always by this model's side. She uses it on her cheekbones, brows, and arches. She smudges it with her finger to get that perfect, yet not so perfect, face that appears like she did nothing at all!

### Jillian Barberie

When she's not on TV, she uses nothing but tinted moisturizer and lip gloss.

### Tyra Banks

When Tyra has a pimple, she becomes creative and changes it into a mole with eye pencil.

### Jennifer Tilly

When nothing is working, this star pulls out the false eyelashes. Tilly claims that with long, natural-looking lashes, her entire face opens up.

### Vivica A. Fox

Petroleum jelly is a beauty staple for Vivica, and she claims that it's a life saver. She uses it to take off those long-lasting lipsticks that are so popular right now. It softens, smoothes, and gently takes away heavy lip stain without drying out her lips.

## Sandra Bullock

Her eyes are her strong point, and she plays them up, muting her cheeks and lips.

She applies her eyeliner in between her lashes rather than drawing a harsh line above her upper lid to maintain that "girl next door" look.

Bullock also keeps her mascara light, applying it only to the tips.

## Nicole Kidman

The key to looking natural and friendly for Nicole is to use no foundation at all.

She uses tinted moisturizer and a little concealer. To copy her look, add moisturizer to your foundation and apply it with your fingers.

To finish her look, she uses a pale pink cream blush to warm up her cheeks and give her that natural, dewy glow for which she is so well known.

## Joan Collins

Here's a star who never leaves the house without makeup and wears sunglasses at the first sign of sun. She claims that she gets her antioxidants at every meal with a glass of red wine.

## Sophia Loren

At sixty-seven, this worldwide legend is still breathtaking. Yes, she claims to eat lots of spaghetti and rub olive oil on her face as moisturizer. But she also gets a tremendous amount of rest (a daily afternoon nap) and quiet workouts. She does forty-five minutes of stretching, abdominal crunches, and a one-hour walk, but is not religious about it.

Her beauty regimen is very simple to follow. Loren adds vitamin A to her eye cream and she uses a simple rosewater toner. You can make your own by making friends with a florist. They have leftover petals galore on a daily basis.

Loren states that any woman can look good if she feels comfortable in her skin. "It's not a question," says Loren, "of clothes or makeup, but an inside sparkle."

### Brigitte Bardot

What's her way of dealing with age? No plastic surgery. She says she gave away her youth and beauty to men and now she is giving her experience and wisdom to her beloved animals.

### Naomi Judd

This fifty-seven-year-old country singer has made a miraculous recovery from Hepatitis C and has wholesome beauty habits. She doesn't eat red meat, and she drinks water constantly.

She also says she gets more sleep than anyone she knows. She must have two hours of quiet time each morning. She also is a strong believer in aromatherapy. She travels in an aromatherapy candle–filled tour bus. Her ultimate bargain beauty secret is applying tons of cheap cold cream all over her skin.

She maintains her size six figure with lots of fresh vegetables.

### Sharon Stone

When it comes to Sharon's hair, she maintains her color with Artec shampoo. She has stopped wearing high heels because it's impossible to feel sexy when your feet are in pain. Her favorite fashion statement is wearing lingerie and pajamas out and about. A favorite outfit is a pair of silk pajamas with slides and diamond earrings.

Sharon doesn't sweat a few pounds up and down and has admitted to a weight range from 115 to 155 on her five-foot-eight-inch body.

### Swoosie Kurtz

At fifty-nine, this actress does yoga four times a week to keep her body flexible and toned. She also claims that it keeps her skin moist and dewy.

### Kim Basinger

Oscar-winning actress and former Breck Girl Kim Basinger is a big believer in colonic irrigation therapy, very popular in Hollywood. She uses It with liquefied wheat grass and a combination of vitamins, minerals, protein, oxygen, and enzymes. She is devoted to detoxifying her body as an age defier and as a form of weight control.

## Isabella Rossellini

The only reason Isabella attends aerobic classes is for the cardiovascular benefits on her heart and her circulation. She prefers stretching and yoga classes for peace of mind.

## Cheryl Tiegs

This former supermodel and *Sports Illustrated* cover girl hikes almost every day. She follows a totally organic diet and practices food combining. One of the reasons her skin looks so fabulous at fifty-six years old is her insistence on sunblock at all times, even under makeup.

## Candice Bergen

Murphy Brown swears that the less makeup she uses, the younger she looks. Her best face is powder, lipstick, and mascara. She also is a believer in facial exercising.

## Kate Capshaw

You've seen her running in movies, and you should know that she runs or hikes four times a week to stay in shape. Her classic wardrobe collection looks elegant and, quite frankly, sexier than those stars who are in their fifties who show too much skin.

## Goldie Hawn

It doesn't seem possible that it's been thirty years since she giggled her way into our living rooms in the comedy show *Laugh-In*. Yet, at fifty-eight, she follows a wheat-free, dairy-free, and sugar-free diet rich in fruits and vegetables. Her absolute favorite ways to stay in shape are power walking, in-line skating, and weight training.

## Michelle Phillips

The former Mamas and Papas singer is a grandmother, and she still looks stunning as she's about to turn sixty. She likes to look good, but has stopped baring her midriff and dresses appropriately. As a former model, she knows that the legs are the last to go, so she plays them up in three-inch heels.

### Mary Lou Henner

*Taxi's* female lead was once twenty-five pounds overweight. She lost it with a fairly stringent diet, which she has chronicled in several books. She claims that she never eats anything that takes a paragraph to describe so she can keep chemicals out of her body. She also relies on lots of tofu and soy products.

### Christie Brinkley

Talk to this model about her diet and you will hear all about her garden because Christie eats according to the season. Having been a vegetarian most of her life, it just makes food sense to her. In the fall and winter, she feeds her family hearty soups filled with vegetables. She prefers this type of eating because it's the kind of food that sticks to her ribs without sticking to her hips and thighs.

What I've always admired about Christie is her refusal to become a waif even when it was "the look." She knows herself and values her health above all else.

She takes ginseng for energy and circulation. It is a stimulant like caffeine, but without any side effects. You can add it tea or take it in capsule form.

### Angelina Jolie

Men and women admire her body, and although she claims she can get too skinny, Angelina does cross train, especially with weights. This optimizes the number of calories burned during a session.

Angelina's favorite snack? She munches on Cheerios throughout the day. She claims they're the best food in the world.

### Jennifer Lopez

Here's the queen of the booty, and she maintains it with deep lunges. You can keep your own from dropping into your leg (what is that, my butt or my leg?) by lunging whenever you're on the phone, brushing your teeth, or during commercials. J.Lo holds eight-pound weights in each of her hands to firm her arms. You can use weights or soda bottles weighed down with sand or salt.

**PILATES** is the rage of the jet set, and **MADONNA** and **LIV TYLER** love it. It's successful because it creates an environment that revs up your metabolism in a way that causes your body to burn more calories even when you're just sitting.

### Pat Benatar

She's still rockin' with the same weight she had in the '80s, a mere ninety-eight pounds. Except now at fifty she has to work at maintaining her weight.

### Missy Elliott

You're seeing less of this leading rapper because she's dropped several sizes. Her method? A low-sodium diet combined with daily walks on the treadmill. Not only does she derive huge physical benefits, she says she feels much more confident.

### Diane Sawyer

When *Good Morning America*'s anchor wanted to lose twenty-five pounds, she turned to green tea. It contains antioxidants and it boosts the metabolism. Sources at the University of Switzerland state that if you drink three cups of green tea a day, you'll burn seventy extra calories.

### Sela Ward

Her forties have been fabulous, and she's reached the pinnacle of her career at this time.

This five-foot-seven-inch beauty hits the Stairmaster and has low-calorie meals delivered to wherever she is working so she doesn't hit the chow line. Her one indulgence is a Krispy Kreme doughnut a day; however, she won't eat one unless she plans to exercise the same day.

### Suzanne Somers

Actress/entrepreneur Suzanne Somers is in her late fifties, and yet people still gasp when she tells them that she has five grandchildren. She has written about her weight struggles and losing parts because she wasn't thin enough. She maintains a diet with low fat and very limited sugar.

### Angela Bassett

Her cheekbones are the best in the business, and her incredibly toned arms rocked in *What's Love Got to Do With It*. She works out an hour a day while watching TV to make the time go by.

### Rene Russo

Another former model turned actress, Rene spent four years of her life in a body cast to combat childhood scoliosis. Because of this experience, she uses the Feldenkrais method, which is an exercise program that improves posture and alleviates pain, as her way of exercising.

Rene uses "Frownies" to keep her face from wrinkling during sleep. If you can't find them in drugstores, make up your own with nonstick adhesive tape. It works similarly. Make an "X" in between your eyebrows.

### Jane Fonda

The former aerobics queen has turned to less strenuous exercising because she says "time is too short." She now practices yoga because it combines spirituality with the body.

Her spirituality is now an important component in her life. She also comments that she never imagined that she would still look so good in her mid-sixties.

### Loni Anderson

WKRP alumna Loni Anderson admits acquiescing to an eye lift because people kept asking her if she was tired. At fifty-eight years old, she has totally reformed her eating habits. Gone are the two doughnuts for breakfast and malted milk balls during the day for quick energy. She now relies on protein for more sustained energy.

### Meryl Streep

Here's an actress you've got to love. She claims she stopped working out three hours a day because she didn't notice any difference. Besides, she has other things to do.

She's fifty-eight years old and a very decent size eight even without it.

### Jaclyn Smith

Former Charlie's Angel Jaclyn Smith is fifty-six and is more health- than weight-conscious today. She's recently undergone successful treatment for breast cancer.

### Susan Sarandon

Here's another star who came from the modeling world. In Paris, she learned to cleanse her skin with milk and continues to do it because it works!

### Raquel Welch

She has married and divorced a pizza entrepreneur fourteen years younger than she is and doesn't worry about it because she's determined to look amazing at seventy.

### Donna Mills

*Knots Landing* star Donna Mills is in her sixties and doesn't give it a second thought.

It's all changed, she says: "The fifties and sixties are now what the thirties and forties used to be." She continues to show off her well-known brown eyes.

# DEBBIE ALLEN CALLS THE FIFTIES THE "SECOND SPRING."

# Model JERRY HALL'S Beauty Rules

❖ She grows her own vegetables because it's the only way she can ensure that she and her family won't ingest any chemicals or pesticides.

❖ Jerry frequents spas for salt scrubs and seaweed wraps.

❖ Olive oil has been a beauty staple since her Texas childhood. Jerry came from a family that didn't have much money, but it was a family of girls so there was lots of experimentation with kitchen beauty. Olive oil is still working for her today. She swears that she doesn't have any stretch marks after four pregnancies because she rubbed her tummy diligently with virgin olive oil.

❖ Jerry insists that a fifty-one-year-old former model should not wear the same clothes as her daughter. Everyone needs some dignity as they age.

### Morgan Fairchild

Morgan loves Botox and admits she's relying on it regularly. She also contends that she and others in their fifties are in better shape than any other generation.

### Lisa Taylor

The former *Vogue* model has hit fifty, and although she weighs ten pounds more than when she modeled, she's perfectly happy and healthy! She eats exactly half of what she used to, recognizing that her metabolism has slowed down with age. Lisa swears that when she looks in the mirror, she can see her spirit showing through her body.

### Beverly Johnson

It's hard to believe that the first woman of color to grace the cover of *Vogue* actually starved herself down to 105 pounds on a five-foot-nine-inch body. She now eats what she wants, gets monthly massages, and claims she's sexier than ever with curves.

Beverly drinks a gallon of water a day and listens to her daughter to keep current.

### Helen Gurley Brown

The original Cosmo Girl and publishing legend still insists on looking her very best as she's about to turn the big 8-0. Her philosophy is to do some kind of exercise each day and not expect applause. It's a form of self respect and a must as we age to fight off jiggle.

A former supplement fanatic, Gurley Brown has gone from forty to fifty supplements a day to just a few. She now takes vitamins E, C, and D, calcium, and a multivitamin.

### Téa Leoni

I love it when I hear about a star who prefers to "do it herself." Such a celebrity is Téa Leoni. This busy mother maintains her blonde highlights by mixing a cup of cool chamomile tea with a little lemon juice, mists her hair with the brew, and then spends time processing it in the sun (about thirty minutes).

### Shania Twain

Besides being an advocate of Bag Balm for her dry skin, this vegetarian chooses only the freshest foods she can find.

### Elizabeth Hurley

How does Elizabeth start her night? She relaxes in a hot bath filled with aromatic oils and a big glass of whiskey.

She attributes her pregnancy weight loss to watercress soup.

### Catherine Deneuve

Another French woman who believes that as we age, we have to make a decision between the face and the derriere. She's very comfortable with a few extra pounds in her sixties and feels it keeps her face from looking old and drawn.

### Patricia Heaton

The beautiful star of *Everybody Loves Raymond* admits her beauty weapon of choice is plastic surgery. She's had her breasts lifted as well as a tummy tuck. Not only do her clothes fit so much better, Heaton says it makes all the difference in how she feels about her body.

# RITA WILSON KEEPS HER SPIRITS UP WITH A PERFECT PEDICURE ALL YEAR LONG.

### Salma Hayek

When Salma goes over her fighting weight of 110 pounds, she simply skips dinner for a couple of nights. She never counts calories because she hates math.

### Kim Cattrall

You've seen more of her body on *Sex and the City* than any of her fellow actresses. She actually gets that body by doing her own housecleaning and walking all around New York.

She also squeezes lemon juice on her French fries to cut out the grease.

### Oprah Winfrey

To get her six glass minimum of water down, she pictures the water flushing the fat cells out of her body.

### Donna Karan

Donna lost a lot of weight with the popular raw food diet. Nothing is cooked over 118 degrees. Fresh is best on this growing food plan.

### Lisa Rinna

This actress keeps her tush tight with butt squeezing. A lot of acting means standing around and waiting for your turn, the perfect opportunity. She even squeezes while going up the stairs.

> "Leaving the house without MOISTURIZER is like walking out the door without UNDERWEAR!"
>
> —Faith Hill

# AGE-DEFYING LEGENDS

**Mae West**, the sexy siren of the thirties, claimed that she kept her skin glowing and her body young by having a daily enema for detoxification.

**Joan Crawford** steamed her face in front of a boiling kettle and then dove into a bowl full of ice cubes to keep it firm and clear.

**Marilyn Monroe** ate spaghetti with a tightly cinched belt so she wouldn't overindulge.

# DYAN CANNON'S FACE EXFOLIANT

- Soak four chamomile tea bags in a quart of water.

- Chill it overnight.

- Wash your face with it in the morning.

- This cleanser has a clarifying effect and cuts through product residue.

> Dyan shares another
> beauty secret:
> take ten to fifteen minutes
> CAT NAPS whenever you can.

# Chapter 5

# AGE-DEFYING MAKEUP

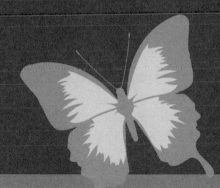

# AGE DEFYING WITH MAKEUP

Cosmetics have the ability to subtract the appearance of years. Or, done incorrectly, they not only add years, but look comical, or worse yet, totally crazy. By now you know what looks good and what needs correcting, what is still hanging in and what's starting to hang.

## COLORS

There's a rule in fashion that if you wore it the first time it came around, don't touch it again. And although that may apply to blue eye shadow, it is not a general rule when it comes to making up. The colors you look good in most likely are the colors you can wear in makeup. If red is your color, you can still stay in the red range, but perhaps a bit more muted.

Whatever you wore boldly now becomes sheerer, just the way the textures of today's cosmetics have become. They're a lot easier to wear.

## MAKEUP RUTS

It can be a combination of fear and laziness. But it can happen at any age. A thirtysomething trying to look like she's sixteen again. A sixty-year-old with ripped jeans and hair extensions doesn't work either. Being in a rut can also be the result of being totally clueless.

Even if you're doing everything right, not changing a color or technique here and there is a sure sign of being in a rut.

## CLUES TO BEING CLUELESS
❖ Still using oil-free foundation. Without oil, foundation creeps into lines.
❖ Stick concealer: it looks too chalky and it cakes.
❖ Sparkling makeup: no matter what it is, it looks like Halloween.
❖ Black eyeliner. Although the aging eye needs definition, it needs to be softer.
❖ Unnatural colors: if you can't find it in nature, lose it.

❖ Pencil-thin eyebrows: the eyebrow is very necessary as we age. It's a mini face lift.

❖ Lip pencil darker than lip color.

❖ Using a concealer that's too light. It must match your foundation; otherwise, it looks like a neon sign pointing to your flaws.

❖ It takes more than five minutes to apply your makeup.

❖ People mistake you for older than you are.

❖ Your makeup rubs off on your clothes.

❖ Your makeup disappears before you're ready to wash it off.

# DON'T

• Use a base with pink undertones.

• Pile on the powder. It makes you look mummified.

# LAYING A FOUNDATION

The purpose of foundation is to even out skin tone. As we age our skin gets blotchier.

The effects of the environment are finally showing up in the form of fine lines and broken capillaries. Skin has becomes dull.

## FOUNDATION MISTAKES

❖ Choosing a color that's too light. Most women think their skin tone is lighter than it actually is.

❖ Trying to bring color to the face with foundation. As we age, we lose color. Unfortunately, it can't be replaced with foundation without looking very unnatural.

❖ Wearing too much. Your foundation should look like you're wearing nothing at all while still providing adequate coverage. Plus, a heavy foundation will only make you look older by drawing attention to every wrinkle.

**Slightly MOISTEN YOUR FINGERS** when applying your foundation. If you use an applicator, such as a sponge, wet the sponge. A little moisture provides a dewy, young surface.

## FOUNDATION CHANGES

Switch to a foundation with a slightly yellow undertone. Don't worry, it won't make your skin look yellow. What it will do is even out blotchiness and redness in the skin and give off a natural finish.

## WHEN IS FOUNDATION **NOT** FOUNDATION?

When it's tinted moisturizer. It just doesn't give enough coverage for aging skin.

To make your foundation look more natural, work it in with your fingers. The heat of your fingers will make it easier to apply, plus you can build up by feel.

## APPLICATION TIPS

Apply moisturizer, then smooth on a firming gel. Leave it on and it will smooth and tighten your skin temporarily under your foundation.

To minimize lines, shower in the morning instead of at night. The humidity will hydrate the skin and allow moisturizer to trap it. This provides a temporary plumping of the skin that should last all day.

Avoid overhead lighting when you apply foundation. It shows every wrinkle and bag. This will encourage over-application. Try to apply foundation near a window, or use lighted makeup mirror with a daylight setting.

Sometimes it's necessary to blend two concealer colors together to get the exact matching shade. While applying concealer, concentrate on the darkest areas first.

Don't forget to conceal the inner corners of the eye, which darken with age.

# SUBTRACTING THE YEARS FROM YOUR EYES

Now is the time to tone it down. No more blue or purple eye shadow. If you're looking for an eye color, take a cue from your eyes themselves. Look at the flecks of color within your eyes. You will find choosing shades similar to those hues will complement your own coloring while making your eyes stand out.

Before applying eye makeup, gently tap eye moisturizer around the eyes with your smallest finger, which will add the least pressure.

Stay away from frosted, bright colors. They make eyes look crepey and old, causing wrinkles and creases to come out and shout at the world.

Choose sheer, neutral colors like cinnamon or a soft rose to give lids a natural flush that mimics young lids.

Line eyes with white pencil just below the lower lids or just inside the inner upper and lower lids to make the eye appear wider and more awake.

Always use an eyelash curler. It's an instant eye lift.

Add a bit of baby oil or petroleum jelly to powdered shadow to instantly look younger and more vibrant.

Highlight your brow bone. It brings attention above the eye, and if you use a shimmering powder it's especially effective.

Open up your eyes by applying a lighter color to your inner eyelids and a darker color on the outside.

Although the aging eye needs definition, a heavy eyeliner can look too harsh. After lining the eye, soften the look by covering the liner with a similar or slightly lighter-colored eye shadow.

# A time-saving option: use a POWDERED EYELINER. Make sure it's got a slightly creamy consistency.

## BROWS

Lift your brows by adding depth and color. Always use short strokes for a more natural look. Hold brows high and in place with brow gel. Nothing polishes a look like a well-groomed brow. It's a frame for the face and takes attention from wrinkles below the eye.

Also, well-groomed eyebrows eliminate aging shadows around the eye.

## APPLICATION TIP:

Tilt your head up slightly when looking
in the mirror and applying eye products.
Don't look down into the mirror.

# IF YOU DON'T HAVE BROW GEL, SUBSTITUTE WITH HAIRSPRAY. YOU CAN SPRAY IT ON YOUR FINGER AND PAT IT ALONG THE BROW, OR SPRAY IT ON A SMALL TOOTH-BRUSH AND BRUSH THE BROW UP.

## WHAT KIND OF BROW?

The brow that will be most flattering is the brow that suits your face. You can actually design your brows to do just that.

A **long face** is balanced with a slightly arched brow. Place the arch outside of the iris, and point the end down toward the top of the ear.

A **square face** requires a centered arch to elongate it. The arch should be above the pupil, and the end should be pointed toward the center of the ear.

A **round face** is best designed with a very high arch placed above the pupil. The end should be short, directed above the ear.

An **oval face** works best with a fairly straight brow, arched just outside the iris, with the end pointing toward the middle of the ear.

**fountain of youth**

**A neutral brow pencil will fill in the brow without looking severe.**

# LIPS

The perfect lipstick can take years away from your face.

It sends the attention to your lips rather than sagging skin and wrinkles.

## WHAT **COLOR**?

❖ Light skin with rosy tones: stay in the range of soft pink shades

❖ Light skin with yellow undertones: choose coral and peach

❖ Medium skin with rosy tones: violet and grape tones are perfect

❖ Medium colored skin with yellow undertones: red shades with blue hues

❖ Dark skin: red/brown/coral tones are most flattering

## fountain of youth

**Bright reds can make lips look even thinner and should be avoided.**

**FULLER** lips are automatically **YOUNGER LOOKING**. You need to "spackle" your lips before applying lip color or else they will show every line. Here's how:

Keep lip color from **BLEEDING** by dipping a cotton swab into foundation and tracing around lips.

**PAT** foundation in with your finger to blend.

Draw a line just **OUTSIDE** your natural lip line with a neutral pencil.

**FILL** lips with pencil.

Finish off with a colored gloss. The **SHINIER** the lip, the younger the look.

**MATTE** lips are aging.

**CHILL THE TIP** of your eye or lip pencil before application, especially in warmer weather for precision.

## **TRICKS** OF THE TRADE

❖ Use curl-enhancing mascara with your regular mascara. It coats the lash in different ways and can correct droopy eyes.

❖ The right shade of taupe powder can work three ways—a shadow, brow filler, and liner when used wet.

❖ Light blush and eye shadow are easier to blend, and they illuminate the skin, making it look younger and more radiant.

❖ Switch to cream blush for a more natural glow. Cream blends in with more ease. Powdered blush just sits on top of the skin, creating an unnatural line.

❖ Place a touch of dark shadow right in the creases of the eyelids to make the aging eye more defined.

## **BODY** TRICKS

To create the illusion of more cleavage, dust bronzer with a large brush in between breasts. This makes the hollow between the breasts look deeper and darker, making the breasts themselves look bigger.

## THE **SMOKY** EYE

A lot of women have been misled and told that they can't wear this look. I actually rely on the smoky eye to take attention away from wrinkles and sagging. It just needs to be softened enough to keep it from looking scary.

# Always **USE BLUSH** with this strong eye treatment to **BALANCE** the face.

# PROBLEMS/ SOLUTIONS

**Small Eyes:** Use a very thin line, as thin as possible.

**Close-Set Eyes:** Line only the outer corners of the eye and never use a pencil or liner that's darker than your own eye color.

**Hooded Eyes:** Pencil should be balanced on both upper and lower eyelids.

**Wide-Set Eyes:** Make them appear closer together by using a darker liner on the inner corners of the eyes. Use a slightly lighter liner on the outer corners.

## GETTING **BRONZING POWDER** TO LOOK NATURAL

❖ Skip the area right under the eye.

❖ Place bronzer on areas of the face that are flat, like the cheeks, forehead, and jaw.

❖ Only use enough to color. You'll know it's too much when it looks powdery.

# Chapter 6

# AGE-DEFYING STYLE

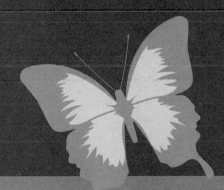

# WHAT IS AGE-DEFYING STYLE?

It's a style that defies rules, especially dictates of past generations.

Maybe there weren't actual *rules*, but there was a definite obligation of certain restrictions, and that made women feel even older and helpless.

## THE **OLD RULES** OF AGING STYLE

Go blonder as you get older? This should not be blanket advice. Some pigments are more complemented by going lighter, but since we lose pigment as we age, you don't want to try to make up for it in your face by going too light.

Long hair does not have to be chopped off just because the candles on your cake are multiplying. Some faces can and need to wear longer hair and actually look more youthful with it. But if your hair looks like a big ball of cotton candy, then you can't do anything else but chop it off.

The zone of length that just doesn't work with aging hair is from below the chin to the shoulder. It's an awkward length on anyone. Either cover your wrinkled neck or give yourself a face lift with a short, stylish cut.

## **DON'T** GO OVERBOARD

You can't be too crazy with style. You can't wear heels so high that you end up looking like an old hooker.

Sneakers look great on kids, but unless you're exercising, you have to watch out for that frumpy look that comes with dressing down.

Big shoulder pads look dated, and they're not coming back. I don't care if they pick your shoulders up. You need to pick your shoulders up by improving your posture. As far as making your hips look smaller, come on. No one ever compliments your hips when you look like a football player.

## PICK A **SIZE**

It makes no sense to have a closet with several sizes of clothing in it. Not only is it not stylish, it's messy and means you are not the driver in your car, sweetie.

## **MAKEUP** IS A STYLE MAKER OR BREAKER

It can make you look like a hussy, or it can make you look years younger. But you simply can't defy age without it.

## STYLE STARTS FROM **INSIDE**

There's a lot more to style than just hair, makeup, and the right clothes. Style is something that is primal in some and a learned skill in others. Age-defying style is a statement that you know what you're doing and want to show what you've got.

Your style represents what you know and think about life. If you go into a group and some interesting music is playing that you've never heard before, you never want to share that "music was so much better" when you were younger. You need to keep that thought to yourself and open up to the ever-changing world.

Learn how to program the VCR and get caught up on the Internet. Computers aren't going away any more than shoulder pads are coming back.

## **DON'T** BE A CLONE

I don't believe in copying anyone's style, especially someone you see on TV.

Especially when it's an anchorwoman. They don't even want to look like that.

Trust me, they've shared this with me many times. Their hair is sprayed beyond recognition so that you will never see it move. Their look is rigid and plastic.

And the colors they wear are TV camera-friendly to match their TV-friendly makeup.

Show off your own style with something new that you yourself have created or found. It could be a new language, a unique style of cooking, or even carpentry.

Research has shown that one of the reasons we age is that we stop exercising the brain.

Keep learning new tricks and you'll never be an old dog. You'll be more interesting, more attractive, younger, and you'll be invited to more dinner parties.

## FAD OR FASHION?

Fashion is not a head-to-toe-trend. Originality is fashion.

Cookie cutter is not fashion.

Inventing your own signature is total fashion. Remember when you were young and you started your own trend? Use something you own in a different way, and you can be ahead of the pack rather than trying to catch up.

Think about the silhouette and not pieces. Figure out what the look is that you're going for. Get the right shape and stick with the basics:

❖ Jeans

❖ Shoes

❖ Bag

You'll look current without looking like you're trying too hard.

Don't go for a piece just because you keep seeing it in the magazines. Get something that just fits you. Make sure that it's not "the" piece to own and is not immediately recognizable in that way.

Those trendy sweat suits, lovely, but who wants to look like a Stepford Wife?

If you've established that a color or fabric works for you, it will work for you throughout the years. If you've always looked great in leather, a little leather is great and youthful. A little leather goes a long way.

Now make adjustments for changing weight, hair color, etc.

## LET IT GO

When a great piece starts to become a joke, then you don't want to be seen in it. Give it up!

# SHOPPING

You can make shopping so much easier and more enjoyable. Some women don't like to shop, especially as they get older. There are ways to save money, look great, and not be obliged to pay for an image consultant.

1. Make friends with a salesperson. She is there to help you and can put things aside for you and have them ready for your visit. Many stores have personal shoppers at no charge. Department stores need the business, so take advantage of this service. Feel free to tell this person that you don't want to hear from her unless she has what you want on sale. That will save you unnecessary trips.

2. Ask to have things selected for you in advance. Though everything will be ready for you in the dressing room, don't feel obligated to buy. Thank the clerk and ask her to try again. If the store has a website, you can pick things out that interest you and give your salesperson the number or description.

3. Magazine advertisers will often include their website or telephone number with their ads. You can call and have them send you the item directly, or they can tell you what stores in your area have it in stock.

4. Write down your size and learn the conversion to French and Italian designers. If you like vintage clothing, be aware that it runs smaller.

5. Bring different sizes into the dressing room. Start with a larger size and work your way down for a perfect fit. Don't try to make something work for you by promising yourself you'll lose a few pounds. It's only the right piece if it fits perfectly.

6. Don't buy something that needs tailoring just because it's on sale. That only makes for closet clutter.

# HOW TO STYLE

## BREAK IT UP

Just because it came together doesn't mean it has to stay together. This especially applies to suits. You'll get more mileage this way and you'll create some fabulous looks.

No matter what your situation in life, you need a suit. You can wear it to a family function or dress it up for evening. You can dress it down for a casual lunch and still look chic by adding a T-shirt.

## MIDDLE AGE **SIGNS**

❖ Someone who's unkempt
❖ Not changing hairstyle for ten years
❖ Not changing eyeglass frames in five years
❖ Not aware of trends
❖ Suntan pantyhose (nobody has that leg color)
❖ Pleated slacks (they don't hide tummies, they're like an arrow pointing to them)

❖ Overly loose clothing
❖ Skirts that fall an inch below the knee (unless you're teaching Sunday School)
❖ Empire waist lines
❖ Hip huggers
❖ See-through fabrics
❖ Cowl necklines (they just droop, and we've already got enough of that)

## OLD FEET INDICATORS

❖ Sensible shoes. Overly sensible shoes just show the world that you've "given it up" for comfort
❖ Tie shoes, unless you're a nun.

The best way to judge the quality of the shoe is to touch it. Leather should feel perfectly smooth, and suede should be very soft. If it's not, then it's not going to be comfortable.

The skin should have no seams and the leather should come from one hide, which ensures a perfect match in hue and texture.

If there's piping or trim, it should look as perfect as a manicure and not ragged.

If the shoe's toe is slightly **UPTURNED** or the shoe **WOBBLES**, that means that the shoe was made really quickly and didn't take the shape it was supposed to. What it means to you is that you're going to be off balance wearing it.

Check out the way a shoe sits on the shelf. If you touch it and it **FALLS OVER**, then you may be falling over in it.

The heel should fit right under the heel of your foot and should give you **GREAT BALANCE** no matter how thin the heel.

If you want heels to be more **COMFORTABLE**, buy a half size larger and put a little toe pad in the front. It will keep your foot back on the heel and keep your toes from pushing painfully into the tip of the shoe.

Before wearing your shoes, take them to a cobbler and have little plastic taps added to the soles at the tip of the toe box if they doesn't already have them. These taps lift the toe just enough to **PREVENT SCUFFING**.

## OLD HAIR

❖ Frosted hair looks like it could never possibly occur in nature. Subtle highlights could.

❖ Tightly curled hair makes you look uptight. Why have a tight permanent when loose is young?

## EYEGLASSES TO AVOID

❖ Big eyeglass frames. Choose a frame without bent bows. They draw your eye down and add years.

❖ Tinted lenses are never stylish.

❖ Don't scrimp on the cost of frames.

❖ Don't go for eccentric or glamorous.

## AGE-DEFYING LENGTHS

Skirt lengths that work are short, to the knee, and to the floor.

If you don't feel comfortable wearing a short skirt, add opaque tights or try a short black skirt with sheer black hose and black shoes—always elegant.

## UNDERSTATED STYLE

It's the easiest look to pull off and the most age defying. With this type of look you can still be comfortable and stylish.

**fountain of youth**

**How Do You Feel About Your Body?**
**It reflects how you choose your style.**

# AGE DEFYING OVER 70

As you head into your seventies, you want to look modern yet distinguished.

Look for the best cut, the best quality, and the best fabric. These three always add up to a great look.

You can add more color if it's a great fit, and wear that fun necklace to "hip" it up.

## MAINTENANCE TIPS

If you're afraid of something shrinking, ask your dry cleaner to use a lower temperature and a shorter cycle than usual.

Ask that your whites and lights be cleaned in new or recently distilled solvent because the white fabric is going to pick up the residue. If you feel the urge, ask to see the solvent so that you can judge for yourself. It should be completely clear.

Have your garment dry cleaned immediately after wearing it. Some fabrics, like silk, don't show their stains right away and the fabric can discolor over time.

Read the labels. Some fabrics are just more resilient. One of my favorites is a wool and polyester mix. Microfibers are easy to maintain. Too much Lycra or spandex will cause fabric to become shiny when ironed.

## AGE-DEFYING CHOICES

Clothing should be not age appropriate but fashion appropriate.

You wear the clothes. They should not wear you.

Think of the style doyennes that you've admired. Jackie Kennedy and Audrey Hepburn are mentioned most often. Their looks showed they were in charge.

**DID YOU KNOW THAT JEANS ARE AGE DEFYING? A heavy denim will lift the derriere and pockets will give the illusion of a rounder butt.**

## PANT CHOICES

**Wide hips:** Darker pants with a boot cut

**Wide waist:** Choose low-rise pants to stretch your torso

**Petite:** Match shirt with belt, pants, and shoes for an elongated look

## TOO **YOUNG**?

If you feel uncomfortable in it, then you'll look uncomfortable.

Trust your intuition.

## TOO **TRENDY**?

Trends are easier to wear when there's a touch of sophistication. A little goes a long way.

## LOOK AT YOUR **BODY**

Know what your assets are and play them up.

Clothes should protect your body, make you feel good, and make you feel pulled together.

## **TOTAL** STYLE

Your style is what people see and immediately perceive about you. You may be falling apart, but you appear totally in control.

# AGE-DEFYING

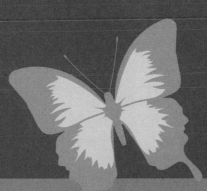

# HEALTH & BEAUTY

Living a healthy lifestyle creates a "younger" life. It's the beauty trick that tops all others.

Changing health habits creates change you can feel and see.

So many myths about aging have been shattered, and there are many ways we can take charge of our health and our beauty as we age.

Women today are turning to a new generation of alternative medicines and food supplements to fight aging and retain their looks.

## LIVE **LONGER** AND **BETTER**

A healthy sense of one's self is an age defier, making us feel and subsequently look better. Those who develop healthy habits such as eating less fat and exercising more have lower stress levels, according to a Yale University study. Such habits also lead to fewer heart attacks and less abdominal fat.

## EXERCISE YOUR **CREATIVITY**

Some of the most remarkable women have done their best work later in life.

Grandma Moses didn't even start painting until she was seventy-eight.

Georgia O'Keeffe won a National Medal of Arts at the age of ninety-seven.

Creativity is key in the anti-aging process.

## BE **TRUE** TO YOURSELF

Those who age well share a surprising trait. They refuse to let others define how they will think or behave. So stop acting your age, put the number away, and you will look a lot better and feel years younger.

## CALCIUM

Women begin to lose more bone mass than they're able to build starting in their thirties.

After that, you need to keep what you have to slow down the loss. Two to three servings a day of dairy or fortified orange juice are a must, more if you are menopausal.

## WATER

It's the forgotten nutrient. It flushes out the system, removes toxins, and helps transport nutrients in the system. If you're continually fatigued and prone to headaches, and there are no medical concerns, consider upping your intake of water. You can also hydrate with decaffeinated teas and fruit to break up the monotony.

## **LISTEN** TO YOUR BODY

It will tell you when it needs fuel. When you are hungry, you need to eat. That said, sometimes we can mistake thirst for hunger. If you continually make healthy choices, you'll minimize your unhealthy cravings. That's because your body has been satisfied with the nutrients it needs.

## SUN HEALTH

❖ Use a moisturizer and foundation with at least an SPF of 15 for extra protection.

❖ Check your sunscreen for a new ingredient called PARASOL. It's recently been approved by the FDA, and is a better blocker of UVA rays.

❖ Look for retinols and alpha hydroxy acids (AHAs) to reduce sun damage. While retinol jumpstarts your skin's process of cell division to break down lines and wrinkles, the AHAs go to work on the top layers of your skin and shed dull layers to reveal younger skin underneath.

# AGE-DEFYING SUPPLEMENTS

## B-COMPLEX

A daily B-Complex supplement that contains folic acid (at least 400 micrograms) has the ability to fend off gray hair. In some cases, a daily dose has literally restored natural hair color.

More naturally, a daily tablespoon of blackstrap molasses, which includes iron and potassium, has also proved important in maintaining hair color.

## NZYME Q10

supplement may offer protection from itive damage. It is found in the highest concentration in the heart, where it helps the cellular mitochondria metabolize fat for energy. It also helps maintain the flexibility of the cell membranes. Coenzyme Q10 levels decline in mitochondria as the body ages, which has led researchers to speculate that mitochondria with less Q10 lose fat less easily.

## DHA & PYRUVATE

The combination of pyruvate and dihydroxyacetone is reported to improve muscle tone, and when added to a healthy eating plan, women lose 37 percent more weight than when they simply count calories. Scientists have found that the combination has the ability to change body composition, so that you're leaner and more toned. It does so by making your cells more efficient at converting food and body fat into adenosine triphosphate, your cell's main source of energy.

## DHEA

DHEA is a hormone that decreases production as we age. Considered the "fountain of youth" hormone, it is reported to help keep everything from brain chemistry to metabolism running young.

One of the side effects that has been reported from DHEA is facial hair growth.

A newer formulation, 7-Keto DHEA, produces more of the benefits without the negatives.

The recommended dosage is 25 to 50 mg daily.

## FOLIC ACID

A British study showed that a daily dosage of 400 micrograms helps to fight heart disease and hardening of the arteries.

## GRAPE SEED EXTRACT

Studies have shown grape seed flavonoids lower blood pressure and boost HDL (artery cleaning) cholesterol. It also helps with wrinkling, sagging, and other signs of aging.

## MILK THISTLE

This supplement helps liver function, which becomes more important as we age.

It also helps to prevent diabetes and is an antioxidant that fights off aging cells.

## PREGNENOLONE

A natural nutritional supplement that is reported to enhance mental alertness and awareness. It also helps joints. Pregnenolone is derived from an extract of the wild yam, which grows in Mexico. The hormone already exists in our bodies, but, as with other hormones, production declines as we age. Proponents of pregnenolone report that it can greatly improve resistance to stress and helps with vision, making colors brighter and clearer.

## VITAMIN K

For years surgeons have been using topical vitamin K to diminish bruising after surgery.

New studies have shown that vitamin K also helps diminish dark circles under the eyes.

# VEINS

Many more women than men seem to suffer from leg veins. They are a progressive problem. Extraordinary results can be achieved with the new vein treatments.

EXERCISE: Moving around is key. If possible, take a brisk walk each day, especially if you're on your feet for long periods.

DIET: Eating a low-salt, high-fiber diet is helpful in vein health. Yo-yo dieting can exacerbate vein issues.

HORSETAIL EXTRACT: In studies, it helped with swelling and increased the skin's defense mechanisms. It is available in creams, or you can buy it as a raw oil at health food stores.

## Don't Forget:

- **Elevate legs at bedtime six to twelve inches above the heart.**
- **Don't cross your legs.**
- **Monitor hormone replacement therapy.**

# AGE-DEFYING TEETH

## GUMS

A study at Emory University discovered that gum diseases such as gingivitis and periodontis speed up the overall rate at which we age because they cause a faster decline of our immune and arterial systems.

If your gums bleed when you brush, your pearly whites are in big trouble. Gingivitis is the first stage of periodontal disease, which can lead to tooth loss and has even been linked to heart disease and stroke. It is caused by buildup of bacteria-infested plaque, which also causes that unattractive yellow tinge. See your dentist immediately for treatment.

Maybe you've had no problem with your teeth, but now you're finding that your teeth have become extra sensitive and are starting to yellow. The reason is that as enamel thins with age, the natural gray color of the dentin, which is the second layer of the tooth, starts to show through. Your teeth also become more sensitive as the enamel thins and little hair-thin fractures develop.

Saliva has anti-bacterial agents, and since its production decreases as we get older, it allows gum disease to form because of the lack of protection.

## BEYOND FLOSSING

Think about eliminating sugar, which is still the main cause of cavities and other tooth problems. Sugar substitutes, surprisingly, can also do damage. So do foods rich in acids like acidic fruits, cola drinks, and foods high in phosphorus.

The proper amount of calcium is important in keeping the jawbone strong.

Vitamin C plays a big role in healthy gums.

## TAKE YOUR TIME AND **TIME** YOURSELF

Two minutes is the minimum amount of time needed to brush properly.

An ultrasonic toothbrush makes it easy since many come with a timing element.

**Wet your toothbrush** before you add your toothpaste, but don't wet your toothpaste. Using toothpaste undiluted makes cleaning more effective.

Add a little **baking soda** to your toothpaste to get rid of plaque and tartar.

## **REVITALIZE** IN YOUR SLEEP

Getting your beauty sleep is a phrase to take literally. It's a sure way to keep your looks and help turn back the clock.

Sleep rejuvenates the body and circulates the nutrients that skin needs for a healthy glow. Although everyone's needs are different, most health experts recommend seven to eight hours a night.

## **SLEEP** HYGIENE

Get into habits that will ensure that you get sound and continuous sleep.

❖ Don't watch TV in bed. The noise increases your alertness, which makes sleep difficult.
❖ Don't check the clock in the middle of the night. It jerks your brain awake.
❖ When you awaken, get up right away so that you don't have a problem falling asleep at night.
❖ Reset your body temperature by raising it before sleep so that your body will automatically lower it. This temperature drop helps

you fall asleep faster and sleep more soundly, according to the Sleep Research Program at McLean Hospital in Belmont, Massachusetts. A nice warm bath can do the trick.

❖ Wearing socks to bed can also induce sleep by lowering your body's core temperature as it draws body warmth to your extremities.

**Check your pillow by folding it in half. If it doesn't open back up again on its own, it's time to replace it.**

# MENOPAUSE CHANGES

Menopause can bring health and beauty concerns that need to be addressed.

With menopause comes a drop in estrogen and consequently all kinds of unpleasant side effects like hot flashes, night sweats, and depression.

## EMPOWER YOURSELF BY LEARNING ABOUT NATURAL SOLUTIONS

**Black Cohosh**

This supplement is a natural way to stave off the effects of menopause. Many women have reported a relatively easy menopause with this over-the-counter supplement.

**Chasteberry**

Packed with mild plant hormones, it is the mainstay of natural menopause treatments in

Europe. Two hundred milligrams daily is reported to relieve hot flashes, fluid retention, nervousness, anxiety, and depression of up to 70 percent of women. It acts on the pituitary gland to help to increase the production of progesterone.

### Red Clover

Doctors say that they've literally erased hot flashes with an extract made from red clover. In a just-released study, forty milligrams in capsule form daily cuts the strength of hot flashes by 70 percent in just four weeks.

Experts claim that mild plant estrogens are the red clover's heat-taming ingredients.

The product name for red clover if you can't find it in a generic form is Promensil.

If you'd like to get red clover naturally, you can get the same amount from a cup of soy milk.

### Evening Primrose and Borage Oils

These are two compounds that contain essential fatty acids to keep skin supple.

### Flaxseed Oil

The healing oil of flaxseed contains both omega-3 and omega-6 fatty acids and is the chemical precursor of the fatty acid EPA. Flaxseed oil is a great remedy for peri-menopausal symptoms, especially skin conditions (itching) and fatigue. It is also reported to lower cholesterol levels and makes insulin more effective while boosting the immune system. You can use flaxseed oil as a salad dressing or as a topping for vegetables, in grains, and in no-heat recipes if you prefer not to take the supplement.

### Ginkgo Biloba

An extract believed to enhance neural synapse connections.

The recommended dosage is 120 to 240 milligrams daily.

### Glucosamine and Chondroitin Sulfate

A supplement combination intended to restore joints and aid flexibility.

The recommended dosage is 1500 milligrams of glucosamine combined with 1200 milligrams of chondroitin sulfate each day. An option is SAMe. Studies indicate that 400 milligrams a day of this amino acid will help rebuild joint cartilage and restore mobility.

## Glutathione

A powerful antioxidant that mops up disease-causing free radicals. It can reverse the damage caused by sun pollution and a less-than-perfect diet. The recommended dosage is at least 150 milligrams in supplement form a day. If you want to get your glutathione naturally, include asparagus in your diet. Just one half of a cup contains 28 milligrams of glutathione. Other good sources include avocados (27 milligrams); spinach, which contains 12 milligrams per cup; and acorn squash, which contains 11 milligrams per serving. Your body rebuilds its glutathione stockpile during sleep, so always make sure you get the necessary amount.

## Soy

Here's another health aid for aging women. Soy represents a safer way to replenish the body's dwindling estrogen supply and is increasingly preferred over the synthetic version used in hormone replacement therapy. According to advocates of soy, it is reported to help with hot flashes and boost cardiovascular health. In numerous studies, soy proteins have been shown to lower LDL (bad cholesterol) by up to 10 percent, according to the Wake Forest University School of Medicine in North Carolina.

You can get soy in tofu, which is an excellent source. Soy milk, roasted soybeans, and shakes made from powdered soy protein and fruit juice are good picks. Researchers recommend a daily dose of 25 grams of soy protein, which equals about a cup of tofu, for best results.

## MENOPAUSE HELP
### FROM JAPAN

In Japan, women never have hot flashes, and the studies point to their diet, which is high in soy protein. Soy contains lots of plant estrogens (isoflavones) compounds that the body can use to offset the drop in natural estrogen and prevent the dramatic surging that triggers hot flashes.

Easy ways to boost soy intake include using soybeans in soups and casseroles or drinking soy milk.

# AGE-RELATED INTIMATE PROBLEMS

## BODY ODOR

Recent research has discovered a substance called DPTA that, when added to deodorants, can cut odor by as much as 90 percent. Look for it in the ingredients list when shopping for a deodorant/antiperspirant. The science behind this is that DPTA deprives bacteria of the iron it needs to reproduce.

## BLOATING AND GAS

Here's a problem that seems to get worse with age. The best way to avoid bloating is to avoid swallowing air. Be careful with carbonated beverages, hard candy, and gum, which can all contribute. Eating too fast is another culprit. Slowing down also decreases belching. Exercise, particularly moving your abdominal muscles, can also help. Make sure you visit your doctor to rule out abdominal diseases, which can also occur with aging.

## FOOT ODOR

Feet have three thousand sweat glands, providing a ready supply of moisture. Combine that with the dark, warm environment of your shoes, and you've got the perfect scenario for foot odor.

To fight foot odor:

❖ Rub an underarm antiperspirant over the bottom of your feet.

❖ Sprinkle your feet with powder, and sprinkle the insides of your shoes with powder.

❖ Let your shoes air out for a day before rewearing.

❖ For a more effective solution, apply a 5 or 10 percent benzoyl peroxide gel to clean, dry feet. This will help kill bacteria as well as prevent foot odor.

If you're prone to foot odor, consider a relaxing foot bath with baking soda. Use at least one quarter cup baking soda with each quart of water.

A wonderful home remedy that is highly effective in fighting foot odor is to sprinkle a little dried sage (yes, right from your spice cabinet) into your shoes before wearing them.

Also effective in reducing odor is to reduce the intake of pungent foods before a social event. Biggest culprits: garlic and onions

If perspiration is extreme in feet or underarms, ask your doctor about the use of Botox to temporarily shut down the sweat glands.

## INGROWN TOENAILS

Another age-related problem; this occurs when the nail on a toe grows or is pushed into the soft tissue behind it or beside it. There is an over-the-counter treatment that is pretty effective called Outgro. If pain is severe or if there is redness, see your doctor. A podiatrist can remove the ingrown part of the nail.

You can prevent ingrown toenails by making sure that you or your pedicurist cuts your nail straight across, and never too short (no deeper than the tip of the toe). Also, avoid tight shoes that press on toenails.

As you age, your foot size may increase. Get measured every few years, especially if your weight has changed.

## TOENAIL FUNGUS

If you see discoloration, thickening, or separating of the nail from the toe bed, you're probably dealing with a fungal infection. It's important to see your doctor for a culture to determine what type of infection you have and the best treatment. Surprisingly, you may be given a prescription to be taken internally along with a topical treatment.

A good preventative measure is to buff your nails on a regular basis, wear proper-fitting footwear, and, if you are prone to fungal infections, use Penlac as a base coat substitute in your pedicure.

## ATHLETE'S FOOT

Soak your feet in water and kosher salt for ten minutes. Use a half cup of salt in two quarts warm water. This will create an environment that is hostile to the fungus. If the infection doesn't clear up within a week, see your doctor for a prescriptive steroid treatment.

A good way to prevent athlete's foot is to thoroughly dry between the toes after bathing or soaking. To ensure that your feet are completely dry, use a blow dryer between toes.

## BAD BREATH

Eighty-five percent of the time, bad breath (or halitosis) is caused by the accumulation of bacteria on the tongue. One very easy way to fight bad breath is to brush your tongue when you brush your teeth.

Don't bother spending needless money on tongue scrapers. Scientists have found that they are not any more effective than simply brushing your tongue at least twice a day.

There are also prescription mouthwashes that neutralize odorous sulphur compounds on contact. On the other hand, a lot of the supermarket/drugstore mouthwashes last only about an hour, and since they contain alcohol, they can dry out your mouth, making your breath worse than ever.

# URGE INCONTINENCE

There are drugs that have been around for years to calm overactive bladders, but most women avoid them due to their unpleasant side effects, which include dry eyes, dry mouth, and constipation. Now there are better drugs. If you have this problem, ask your doctor about Ditropan XL, which is reported to cut attacks by as much as 85 percent. In one study, it actually cured 43 percent of the subjects overnight. Another new option is Detrol, which calmed excitable bladders in 52 percent of women studied.

# Chapter 8

# AGE-DEFYING NUTRITION

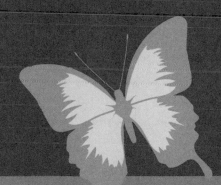

# INSIDE/OUTSIDE BEAUTY

The link between internal health, beauty, and anti-aging is becoming more and more clear. You eat it, and you'll end up wearing it. The intent is to wear clearer, more radiant skin, and a firmer, leaner body. There is no better ally to fight aging than the right foods.

## GET OUT OF YOUR FOOD RUT

Stop fixing those big, stick-to-the-rib meals and switch to mini meals.

Drink a glass of ice water before every meal. You will be fuller, and you may discover that what you mistook for hunger was really thirst.

## SNACK A LITTLE

Save enough calories to snack three times a day to keep an aging metabolism revved up.

## LEAVE A LITTLE FAT

For younger-looking skin, it's necessary to eat enough essential fatty acids.

This is not the fat on a steak, but in salmon, flaxseed, sunflower seeds, avocados, and nuts.

## MODERATE ALCOHOL CONSUMPTION

You've heard that wine has antioxidant value and that is very true. Just look at Jack Lalanne, fitness guru to many generations, who says that the key to his longevity is two glasses of red wine every day. Or ageless beauty Joan Collins, who has a glass of wine at each meal. But too much alcohol dilates capillaries and can cause skin to flush. Plus, too much alcohol can disrupt sleep, cutting into your most necessary beauty aid.

## fountain of youth

**If your skin is prone to rosacea, avoid food triggers like spicy foods, chocolate, and hot drinks.**

## GET ENOUGH CALCIUM

To prevent osteoporosis and keep teeth strong and healthy as we age, it's necessary to get at least 1,000 milligrams of calcium daily up to the age of 50 and 1,200 milligrams after the age of 50.

**GOOD SOURCES OF CALCIUM ARE FAT-FREE MILK, CALCIUM-FORTIFIED ORANGE JUICE, AND LOW FAT HARD CHEESES.**

## CUT DOWN ON REFINED SUGARS

They provide a dramatic energy high and then a drop, creating tension and stress, which can contribute to aging.

## CALM DOWN ON CAFFEINE

A little caffeine is actually good. It gets your metabolism going. Caffeine has even been shown in research to elevate mood, though too much creates stress and jitters. Too much can also bring you crashing down, making your levels of insulin (the fat-storing hormone) go up, making it harder to keep weight off.

## EAT YOUR FRUITS AND VEGETABLES

Studies have shown that people who are 20 percent or more above their ideal body weight generate substantially more free radicals than those who are close to their ideal weight.

One way that you can fight back, according to these studies, is to fill your plate with colorful, high-fiber fruits and vegetables. They are the foods that have the highest levels of antioxidants and produce the fewest free radicals when they're digested. Another benefit is that they will induce weight loss.

## RED MEAT AND CHOLESTEROL

Although red meat has received its fair share of bad publicity in regards to health, studies indicate eating lean red meat five times a week can slash artery-clogging "bad" cholesterol levels by 12 percent. Red meat is rich in stearic acid, a compound that helps control cholesterol levels and keep arteries clear. A Harvard study found that women who eat the most protein are 29 percent less likely to develop heart disease.

## EGGS

Also helping in aging is the much-maligned egg. New studies have discovered that eggs are rich in lutein, a pigment that prevents arteries from clogging and protects against the blockages that lead to heart attack and stroke. Studies further indicate that people who have the most lutein in their blood have the clearest arteries.

## CHEESE

The fat in cheese contains conjugated linoleic acid, shown to boost the body's fat-burning furnace and increase muscle.

## FOOD RULES

❖ Eat breakfast within an hour of getting up to get your metabolism going.
❖ Eat five smaller meals instead of three big ones.
❖ Make breakfast your biggest meal and dinner your smallest. Metabolism slows at night, meaning that this is when your body is most prone to storing fat.

## FOODS THAT TURN BACK TIME

**Asparagus**
Each serving provides folic acid and other age-fighting nutrients.

### Beets

Full of antioxidants for the skin and detoxifiers that target the liver.

### Blueberries

Contain more antioxidants than any other fruit or vegetable. Researchers at Tufts University state that just one cup of blueberries daily, especially wild blueberries, quadruples anti-aging compounds that can keep wrinkles away. Dr. James Joseph of the Jean Mayer USDA Human Nutrition Research Center on Aging at Tufts University did a study in which "geriatric rats" regained youthful characteristics after being fed a diet high in blueberries.

### Bran

Keeps your digestive system regular, preventing age-related constipation and hemorrhoids.

### Citrus fruits

Packed with vitamin C to help bolster your immune system. Vitamin C has been linked to smoother skin and reduced risk of arthritis.

### Cherries

Contain quercetin, a powerful antioxidant that fights inflammation.

### Garlic

Cleanses pores from the inside out, lowers blood pressure, reduces cholesterol, and contains anti-bacterial/anti-fungal properties.

### Kiwi

Contain the most vitamin C of any fruit. Vitamin C is key to maintaining smooth skin.

### Romaine lettuce

Contains twice as much folic acid, six times more vitamin C, and eight times more beta-carotene than other lettuces.

**Sweet Potatoes**

Contain 20 percent more fiber and fewer calories than regular potatoes. Contain 86 percent more potassium and zinc. It's considered to be a real beauty food. An entire sweet potato has only 115 calories.

**Tomatoes**

Researchers at the University of Illinois at Chicago state that tomatoes and tomato products are nature's number-one source of lycopene, an antioxidant that fights tissue-damaging free radicals.

**Yogurt**

Full of calcium and one of nature's oldest health foods to fight high blood pressure. Look for yogurt thickened with live cultures rather than gelatin.

**Olive Oil**

Taken internally, olive oil stimulates metabolism, promotes digestion, and lubricates membranes.

Australian scientists discovered that people who eat a lot of olive oil are much less prone to wrinkling and sagging than those who eat a lot of butter. Olive oil protects the collagen, elastin, and other underlying support structures of the skin. Try to have at least a tablespoon of olive oil in your diet each day.

If you've been buying regular olive oil, switch to extra virgin. Extra virgin is made from the first pressing of the olive and contains higher amounts of antioxidants.

## AGING AND YOUR BLOOD SUGAR

Your glucose levels can determine if you're getting old before your time. If glucose levels are high, dangerous sugar molecules can attach themselves to collagen and elastin proteins, which can hasten the aging process in every part of the body.

You can lower your glucose levels and your weight by cutting down on refined sugars.

## EAT YOUR WAY TO BETTER HAIR

Here are three natural ingredients to include in your diet that will help with hair growth, volume, and shine:

**Niacin**, found in chicken, tuna, and whole wheat foods, delivers nutrients to the hair follicles.

**Omega-3 fatty acids**, found in fresh fish, canola oil, and walnuts, increase volume and shine.

**Zinc**, found in red meat, shellfish, and dark meat chicken and turkey, promotes hair growth and strengthens hair strands.

## FIGHT WRINKLES WITH KETCHUP?

Yes, just a dollop of ketchup a day can protect your skin from sun damage and premature aging. A German study was done that found those who ate just two servings of carotene (which ketchup is high in) had much less skin damage than those who didn't.

## GOOD FOODS/BAD FOODS

**Fast Foods**

They can play havoc with aging, and, worse yet, they are so quick and convenient. Soda, combo meals, super size, double anything are major culprits.

Get grilled meat whenever you can, and skip the soda in favor of water. More and more fast food restaurants are now providing calorie counts. Don't hesitate to ask for a low-calorie alternative.

**Fruit Drinks**

There's something so wrong with some of these drinks being called "fruit" anything when most of the drink is sugar and as little as 10 percent is fruit juice.

A better choice is pomegranate juice, available at health food stores and natural supermarkets. UCLA researchers report this juice has more than five times the polyphenol content of its contender, green tea.

Polyphenols are among the most powerful anti-aging compounds available. They have the ability to absorb skin-damaging free radicals like a sponge.

### Go Light on Salt

After fifty, women may become more sensitive to salt, which may raise blood pressure and cause fluid retention.

### Strengthen Your Teeth

Oranges, lemons, and other citrus fruits contain bioflavonoids that strengthen bones and teeth. The vitamin C in citrus also aids the absorption of calcium to reduce the risk of osteoporosis.

### Eat Fiber at Every Meal

If you double your daily fiber intake, your body will absorb fewer calories.

### Detox

It's becoming more and more popular in the fight against aging. Detoxing stops cravings, sheds water weight, restores the liver's natural fat-burning power, and jumpstarts aging metabolisms.

There are different approaches to take with detoxing. It can range anywhere from a one-day fast to actual detoxing soups that you can live on from anywhere to two days to an entire week. You can also use herbs to detox.

### Apple Pectin

Cleans toxins and waste from the body, allowing calories to be burned more efficiently.

### Cayenne Pepper

Stimulates metabolism by having a heating effect on the body that stimulates circulation, opens the pores, and promotes detoxing through perspiration.

### Flaxseed

Power cleans toxins and waste from the body and acts as an appetite suppressant.

**GInger Root**
Stimulates your metabolism and prevents water retention.

**Parsley**
A natural diuretic.

**Peppermint**
Stimulates circulation and opens pores.

**Psyllium Husk**
A metabolism booster and natural laxative.

# DETOXING SOUP RECIPES

## Cleanser

Combine one quarter cup each chopped red cabbage, carrots, yellow squash, and celery.
Add one teaspoon chopped parsley and one cup water.
Bring to a boil.
Cover and simmer until vegetables are tender.
Puree until smooth.

Makes one serving (thirty calories).

## Metabolism Booster

Combine one half cup each chopped apple and zucchini, one quarter cup avocado,
and one teaspoon each fresh basil and fresh cilantro.
Add one cup of water and a dash of curry powder.
Bring to a boil.
Cover and simmer until tender.
Puree until smooth.

Makes one serving (ninety-five calories).

## Fat Blocker

Combine one third cup each chopped broccoli, zucchini, and rutabaga.
  Add one chopped onion, one teaspoon cilantro, and one cup water.
  Bring to a boil.
  Cover and simmer until tender.
  Puree if desired.

  Makes one serving (thirty-three calories).

# Chapter 9

# AGE DEFYING ON A BUDGET

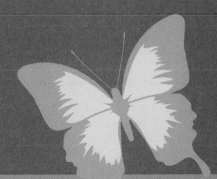

Aging well is not a privilege of only the very rich. There are inexpensive approaches and products that will make a definite difference.

## LASER ALTERNATIVES

Massage vitamin K into your age spots. As few as six applications will fade them away.

Use 2 percent hydroquinone (fading cream) to get rid of age spots and skin blotchiness.

## GET BACK THAT **BABY SKIN**

Exfoliation is the key to shedding the years. Nothing perks up a tired complexion faster. Exfoliating also boosts circulation.

Exfoliate every day with vitamin C or ester C powder. You can find it with the vitamins. Wet the powder with a small amount of water and gently scrub face and hands. This will provide more power than vitamin C scrubs, and the savings are incredible.

## DO YOUR OWN **FACIAL**

Steaming your face over boiling water may be free, but it can burn the face. Heat water until it simmers and then pour it into a metal bowl. Squeeze a fresh lemon into the water.

Lean over the bowl and drape a towel over your head for five minutes.

Soak a cotton ball with a teaspoon of lemon mixed with witch hazel (found in drugstores) to remove impurities.

Finish off with a moisturizer application and a massage. Starting at the collarbone, run your finger lightly over your throat with a hand-over-hand movement, up and out.

Then, place the back of both hands under your chin and gently tap your fingers against your chin, working out from the center and upward toward your earlobes.

Place your index finger gently at the corner of your mouth by the line that runs from the side of the nostril. With the fingers of your other hand, gently work the skin in circles, upward and outward.

## PLUMP UP YOUR **LIPS**

Apply cinnamon oil to your lips. It will temporarily make them fuller by bringing blood flow to the area. Check for sensitivity by applying on your wrist first.

Neutral colors like cinnamon, peach, and light plum make thinning lips look plumper.

## CHANGE YOUR **BROW** SHAPE

By changing your brow shape, you can make your face look thinner and younger.

❖ Create a high arch. Draw a high triangle above the outside corners of the pupil with a white pencil. Pluck the marked areas.

❖ Fill in sparse brows for a younger look. Use neutral colored shadow, such as taupe. Apply with an eyeliner brush.

## GIVE YOURSELF AN **EYE LIFT**

An eye lift can make you look ten years younger and is one of the most popular procedures in cosmetic surgery. You can use a few little tricks of the trade to get the same effect with little or no money.

❖ Make dark circles disappear with a perfect matching concealer. It's the foundation that has settled in the cap. The thicker consistency makes it the perfect match.

❖ Turn you eyelash curler into a mini curling iron by dipping it in warm water for ten seconds. Your eyes will perk right up.

❖ Make your eyes look more lifted by applying a light cream-colored shadow on the inside of the eye to the corner of the nose.

## DITCH THE **POWDER**

Blot your face with a separated tissue instead of powdering. Powder settles into every line and crease, making them more visible and making you look years older.

## **TRAIN** YOUR EYES

Placing adhesive tape over furrows will train the eye muscles to stay relaxed. It's very important to apply the adhesive while you sleep so that the tape will prevent nighttime unconscious wrinkling, which is uncontrollable without the tape. Apply the adhesive in an "X" between eyes.

The best tape to use is surgical tape since it takes less effort to pull it off every morning.

When it comes to **POWDER PRODUCTS** like eye shadows, there's almost no difference between inexpensive brands and their high-priced counterparts. It's all about shades, colors, and often pigment. I prefer to use less pigment for a more natural look.

# BUDGET BODY

## EXERCISE

Moving your body is like taking an anti-aging pill. You don't need to join a gym, and doing something you love will ensure that you'll look forward to exercising rather than dreading it. Walking, gardening, and heavy housework all strengthen heart, lungs, bones, and muscle. They boost the immune system and keep you looking and feeling younger.

## BREATHE DEEPLY

Scientists are discovering that meditation helps keep us wrinkle free and healthy.

One study found that those who meditated for five years were fifteen years younger biologically than those who didn't. No, you don't need a mantra or a special room, just a quiet place and a few minutes a day to breathe deeply and relax those wrinkles away.

## STRETCH YOURSELF YOUNG

This simple move increases circulation, infuses the body with energy, and erases furrows from the face.

Start in a lowered push up position with hands in line with shoulders, feet hip width apart.

Exhale and push up with your arms, also lifting your buttocks up until you're in an upside down V, shifting weight onto your heels. Hold to the count of ten, inhale, and return to start position.

Repeat five times.

## FACE-LIFTING EXERCISES

So you say you can't afford a face lift? Or you just don't want to go under the knife?

There are gentle exercises to help your face stay youthful. Always remember to be careful, and never stretch the skin.

❖ Start to smile, and then stop it in mid smile without parting your lips. Try to force the corners of your mouth upward, but don't let them rise. Repeat ten times.

❖ Stick out your tongue as far as you can and try to reach your nose. Even though you won't be able to, just by trying you'll tighten the muscles in the center of your neck and define your jaw line. Repeat ten times.

❖ Further tighten up the jawline by sticking your bottom lip out as far as it will go. Hold to the count of five. Relax and repeat seven times.

❖ Place your index finger gently at the corner of your mouth along the line that runs to the side of your nostril.

❖ With lips closed, try to blow air out, filling your cheeks and around the mouth with air. Hold at the fullest point for a count of five. Repeat five times.

## SPRAY ON THE PAST

Nostalgic scents like cinnamon, orange, and vanilla evoke memories and make us feel younger.

## HIDE LINES WITH BANGS

If you're bothered by a lot of forehead lines and don't want to spend a lot of money on Botox, consider bangs. Keep them long, wispy, and textured for a modern look.

## SUDS YOUR SCALP

You can save money and time by shampooing only the roots of your hair. Too much cleansing strips aging hair of its natural oils, causing breaking and splitting.

## REPAIR YOUR HAIR

Clarify your hair inexpensively by spritzing on a mixture of three tablespoons of water and one tablespoon of lemon juice. Apply to just-shampooed damp hair and let it sit for twenty minutes. The citric acid will clean your hair of any residue and will make it shine.

## COLOR AWAY THE YEARS

Warm highlights around the face and at the crown brighten your complexion and draw the eye upward, diverting attention from wrinkles. Plus, highlighting only around the face will cost a lot less than a full head of highlights.

## COLOR YOUR OWN HAIR

Yes, you can get great do-it-yourself hair if you go slowly, don't do anything too drastic, and read the directions. Oh, and if you can grab a friend to help, it will be a lot easier.

Find a friend who may want you to reciprocate, and you've got it made.

1. Prep your skin with petroleum jelly. When hair color gets on skin, it's hard to get off and makes the hair job look messy.
2. Don't go too dark or too light. If you have to wear more makeup to make your color

work, then it's the wrong color. Color is meant to make your face look more vibrant, not drained.

3. Buy two different colors. Hair around the face is usually lighter and brighter, yet most women usually pour one color all over their heads. The second, slightly lighter color goes on at the end of the coloring around the face to create a more professional look.

## RETOUCHING

It isn't necessary to color the entire head each time. Plus, it just causes hair ends to get increasingly drier.

Apply hair conditioner to the ends of your hair. Apply color to roots, allow it to process, and then refresh the ends by working the formula right over the conditioner and let develop for the final five minutes.

## RESCUE WORK

If you don't feel that your hair color is quite right, dilute the color with an equal amount of shampoo.

Lather, then let sit for five minutes.

Rinse.

You'll be adding just a shimmer of color with shine.

# Chapter 10

# AGE-DEFYING HAIR

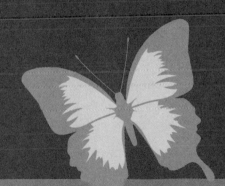

# REVERSING THE STRANDS OF TIME

Your hair, along with everything else, ages. The hair shaft begins to lose volume, becomes drier and more fragile. Hormonal changes will cause hair strands to gray. Your hair will also begin to feel much coarser.

## THINNING

Calcium is beginning to build up in the follicle. This restricts the growth of the hair to the shaft. The growth cycle is changing, and more follicles are now resting.

## CHOICES

There's a lot that can be done. A new and refreshing hair color, a more flattering cut, and some simple restorative techniques are a few options.

A new **HAIR COLOR** can perk up pigment, which fades with age. Go a little lighter, especially around the face.

**SHINE** is young and matte is old, even when it comes to hair. There are shine-enhancing products on the market, and your stylist can give you a shine treatment.

A wash-in **HAIR GLOSS** can enhance your natural color, or you can purchase a tinted color for extra oomph!

Don't let your age define your hair length. Just because you've seen your fortieth or fiftieth birthday, you don't have to cut your hair. Some women look great in short hair and some cannot carry it off. You really don't need to have hair much past your collarbone. Past the collarbone drags the face down.

# HAIR **DON'TS**

### Short bangs
They're not flattering and look like you're trying too hard to be hip.

### Barrettes, headbands, etc.
Use style-control products instead.

### High heat exposure
Your hair is too fragile to do the daily flat iron routine.

### Too many chemicals
The good thing about graying is that you don't have the dark roots that have to be addressed, so you can lessen the abuse to your follicles.

### Waist-length hair
Sorry Rapunzel, Woodstock has long gone.

### Bulky, fluffy hair
Your hair should look sleek and smooth, not like cotton candy. A study done at Yale University showed that people with frizzy hair are perceived to have lower intelligence.

### Rough towel drying
Stop beating up your hair. Plus, you're creating tangles that will require pulling to get out.

### Overdrying
Frying your hair does not make it behave.

### Combing after towel drying
It causes hair to break. If you need to comb at all, apply a leave-in conditioner and use a wide-tooth comb. All you really should do is squeeze out excess water.

### All one color

It looks fake, especially if it's dark hair. Always break up color with two or three subtle highlights.

### Black, black hair, especially blue/black

It throws shadows into skin lines. Go at least a shade lighter than you were five years ago.

### Dark ends

The ends of your hair are more porous and soak up more color. To prevent this, rub a small amount of leave-in conditioner into the ends of your hair before coloring.

# GRAY DECISIONS

You can embrace the gray, let it stay, or, if you prefer, get rid of it. Some women were born to have this color, but it can make others look washed out.

Gray hair does take extra care to help it look its best.

❖ Don't use high heat on gray hair. It will singe and turn yellow and brassy.
❖ Don't overuse relaxers. Gray tends to be coarse.
❖ Don't use colored gel or styling products. Gray hair absorbs every color.

When you start seeing gray hairs, don't pull them out. As you age, your hair is thinning and you need all the hair you can find. Instead, use a gentle vegetable color. It adds body without lightening the roots.

Blonde hair over gray can be tricky. Be sure to establish a base color that's not gray before applying blonde or blonde highlights.

If your hair is only one-third gray, you probably only require a semi-permanent rinse. It covers gray while boosting shine and looks very natural.

Make sure you are getting plenty of protein and vitamin B-rich foods in your diet, which can help slow down the graying process. Foods like turkey, bananas, sweet potatoes, and spinach are all good choices.

# TRICKS AND TIPS

## CHANGE YOUR SHAMPOOING SCHEDULE

Washing every day strips hair of natural oils, leaving it even more dry and fragile. There's no need to wash hair more than three times a week. Giving it a rest will allow natural oils to build up again and replenish hair. Be sure to use a moisturizing shampoo and conditioner. A leave-in conditioner is especially helpful for aging hair.

A few strategically placed **highlights** at the crown and sides of the face give it a lift.

**Brightening** the face gives the skin radiance and takes away dull or ashy tones.

Hair with more **volume on top** also brings your face up. Longer hair should be **layered** for more height and fullness. Hair should never be too structured or tight. Free hair without being messy is the look of youth.

**Bangs** hide deep forehead wrinkling. The best bangs are a bit longer on the sides. That said, keeping hair away from the face can also act as an instant face lift. Keep experimenting.

**Downplay laugh lines** by having your stylist trim hair just below the jawline to draw the eye away from the sides of the face.

The day before you plan to color, mash three aspirin into your shampoo to **dissolve product buildup** that might cause uneven coloring.

**Build volume** with a "body" massage. Turn your shampoo into a treatment by deeply **massaging your scalp**. Massage boosts circulation and helps to bring oxygen, protein, and vitamins to the scalp, promoting hair growth.

Protect hair from **sun exposure**, which weakens and dries hair further. Buy a large, fun hat and look for products with sunscreen protection.

A deep **side part** gives instant life to your hair, especially if you switch it over to the opposite side.

Keep your haircolor from **fading** by installing a showerhead water filter that blocks chlorine.

Women of color can age defy their hair by leaving **relaxing products** in for at least five minutes less. Chemically treated hair absorbs color more quickly as it ages.

## SUPPLEMENTS

Silica tablets, sold at drugstores and mass merchandisers, can help stop hair loss. They are sometimes called the hair/skin/nails vitamin.

Take 500 to 1,000 milligrams of primrose oil a day to generally aid to the health of your hair and enhance its shine.

# WORKING WITH YOUR STYLIST

By now you probably have a good idea about how you like to look. You're probably comfortable with your style—it gets you out the door quickly, and you've been doing it for a while. It's time to re-evaluate your look, be daring, and try something new without going completely out of your comfort zone.

Before getting a new cut, go to a store where they sell wigs. Bring a friend with you and have pictures taken in a few styles and colors. Bring these pictures, along with pictures from magazines of styles you like, to your stylist. It's one thing to describe a look, another to see it. Pictures say a lot. Plus, you need to see yourself with your dream style to see if it will work when you're awake.

The change can be minor, like changing a part or adding bangs or a few extensions.

But to defy age, change is good. If you are guilty of "helmet head," overstyled, and over-processed hair, change is a must.

Now is the time for more maintenance and paying for a good service. The better the cut, the easier your hair will fall into place. Your style will remain bouncy and healthy.

## HAIR WEAVING

It's a procedure that more and more women are exploring to get the volume of youthful hair. It takes money and time, but the results can be amazing.

# For hair coloring, go to a salon that uses ROLLER-BALL HEATING LAMPS.

# HAIR RECIPES

## Hair Reviver

Mix one half teaspoon olive oil with three tablespoons of hair conditioner.
Heat in microwave for ten seconds.
Smooth over hair and comb through.
Let set for fifteen minutes and shampoo out.

## Volume Builders

• Add a few drops of peppermint oil to one teaspoon olive oil.
Massage into dry scalp before shampooing.

• Add a teaspoon of rosemary to two tablespoons shampoo.

• Look for hair products containing dimethicone or dimethicone copolyol.

• Drink one to three cups of green tea a day. Green tea Inhibits enzymes that cause hair loss.

## Color Protector

After a color treatment, wet your hair with a vinegar-based salad dressing.

The vinegar will seal the cuticle to lock in color and the oil will add moisture to your hair.

Leave on for fifteen minutes.

Rinse with cool water.

# PRODUCT RECOMMENDATIONS

## VOLUMIZING **SHAMPOO**

Look for the ingredient polyquaternium-10. It gives body to the hair and acts as a detangler.

## VOLUMIZING **STYLERS**

Look for copolymers, which hold your hair away from your scalp. One that is common to drugstores is polyquaternium-4.

## **LOW-PH** PRODUCTS

The last thing you need are harsh, drying detergents. There are actually some hair shampoos that share factories with carpet shampoos. Enough said.

**TIP:** pH balanced doesn't really mean much. Look for **low pH** on the label.

## **AMINO** ACID

Look for this ingredient to balance the moisture in your hair.

# Chapter 11

# AGE-DEFYING FAST FIXES

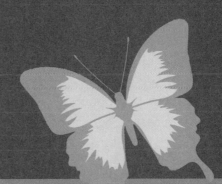

Everybody has beauty emergencies, no matter what our age. If something can go wrong, it does, and it's usually at the worst moment, such as when we're headed out the door to something important.

# FIGHT FATIGUE

You can look and feel refreshed in just sixty seconds, no matter how tired you are feeling at the end of the day. When you're tired, you look older.

## ACUPRESSURE

Gently press your temples, the bridge of your nose, or just below your bottom lip with your fingertips. It balances the body's energy field and replaces feelings of listlessness with vitality.

## PEPPERMINT

Slick a light coating of peppermint oil over your lips. Peppermint oil opens up your sinuses so you can breathe in more oxygen and regain energy.

## TAI CHI

Sit in a chair with your feet flat on the floor and your hands in your lap, palms facing upward. Breathe in deeply and raise your arms above your head, palms facing the sky.

Exhale, and bring your arms parallel to the ground.

Repeat.

## OXYGEN BOOST

Breathe deeply in and out for sixty seconds to send oxygen to every cell in your body.

Breathe so that your diaphragm expands as you inhale and deflates as you exhale.

# PROBLEM NAILS

### RAGGED CUTICLES

Get rid of excess cuticle with Alka-Seltzer. Soak a couple of tablets in a cup of warm water. Massage in with a toothbrush and rinse thoroughly

### PEELING NAILS

Rub on a glycolic acid face cream. It will act as an exfoliant to slough off the roughness.

### NAILS THAT **WON'T GROW**

Nail growth slows down as we age. Gelatin is enriched with nail-building amino acids.

Take a packet of unflavored gelatin (available at grocery stores) and mix with a tablespoon of petroleum jelly. Massage into nails each day.

If possible, do this in the evening and wear cotton gloves overnight.

**MAKE NAILS LOOK LONGER IMMEDIATELY BY APPLY A TOP COAT OF TRANSLUCENT PEARLY NAIL POLISH OVER YOUR NAIL COLOR. IT REFLECTS LIGHT TO VISUALLY LENGTHEN YOUR NAILS.**

## DISCOLORED NAILS

Use whitening toothpaste on yellowed areas or soak your nails in a couple of denture tablets and warm water.

## BROKEN NAIL

1. Clean off the broken nail so you can see what you need to fix. Dip your nail into a bottle of polish remover to avoid ruining your other nails.
2. Carefully swab it down with a tissue or cotton ball.
3. Trim only enough of the nail so that no trace of the split is left.
4. If the split has entered the nail bed, tear off a tiny scrap of tea-bag paper.
5. Dab the crack with super glue and place the tea-bag paper on top.
6. Let it dry for five minutes and then buff the break with a nail buffer.
7. Apply two coats of polish.

## Fix chipped nails with washable magic marker if nail polish is not available.

# SKIN EMERGENCIES

## ROSACEA

Dab it with maple syrup.

Maple is an anti-inflammatory emollient that calms and soothes skin.

Rinse after two minutes.

Press undiluted dandruff shampoo on with a gauze pad for sixty seconds.

Rinse with cool water.

## MENOPAUSAL **ACNE**

Apply an ice cube to bring the swelling down.

Zap it with tea tree oil. It won't dry out skin and you can dab powder right over it.

Tea tree oil has anti-viral properties that zap blemish-causing bacteria on contact.

## BROKEN **CAPILLARIES**

Take a small liner brush and dip into foundation. Paint over the capillaries.

This renders them invisible. If you find that your foundation is too moist to cover the capillaries, then first dip into the foundation and then dip into a dot of powder.

## **RUDDY** COMPLEXION

Mix a small amount of blue eye shadow with powder to cover ruddy spots.

Blue has neutralizing power and, when mixed with the powder, does not show up as blue on the skin.

## **SCORCHED** SKIN

Combine one half cup mayonnaise with one tomato, one cucumber, and half a mashed avocado.

Puree in a blender until smooth.

Apply to skin and allow to air dry.

Rinse well and moisturize.

## SUNBURN

Gently rub apple slices on the affected area for fifteen minutes.

Rinse.

Spritz your face with cooled chamomile tea.

Rub shimmery bronzer on your face to neutralize the redness with sparkling flecks.

Pat sheer highlighting cream along the tops of the cheekbones to the temples.

## FACIAL **BLOAT**

To quickly ease puffy skin, press above eyebrows and circle in toward the center of your forehead. Then, gently circle out at cheekbones and temples.

Circle out on chin.

This motion stimulates blood flow to redistribute fluid that can cause swelling.

Lie over the side of your bed, face down, and count to sixty.

## FACE **FIRMERS**

Combine one raw egg with a teaspoon each of honey and almond oil. Apply to face for ten minutes and then rinse.

Take the egg white out of the egg and place wherever you want to lift the skin (around eyes, mouth). Do not move a muscle until it dries.

Apply makeup. Your makeup should go right over the egg white without disturbing it.

## **PUFFY** EYES

Cucumber helps drain the fluids that pool beneath your eyes often caused by lack of sleep.

1. Cut a couple of cucumber slices. Lie on your back and press the juice of the cucumber into the puffiness for ten minutes.

2. Soak two black tea bags in warm water and let steep until cool. Place over eyes for ten minutes.

## **RED** NOSE

Apply foundation mixed with green eye shadow. The color green cancels out redness.

Finish off with a light dusting of powder.

## **DARK** CIRCLES

Add yellow eye shadow to foundation.

Use a brush or your ring finger and apply the foundation over moisturizer.

Start beneath your eye's inner corner and spread above outer corner, including the area under the lower lashes.

Set with pressed powder.

Apply makeup as usual.

## **TIRED** SKIN

Rev up circulation and energize your complexion by using menthol as a skin cleanser.

Use a damp washcloth and apply in a circular motion.

Menthol boosts blood flow and gives an immediate healthy pink flush.

Rinse with cool water.

# MAKEUP

## NO TIME

If you have only a minute to throw on some makeup, under-eye concealer, pencil at the outer corners of the eye, and sheer lip gloss will get you out the door.

If you have five minutes to spare, even out blotchiness with cream-to-powder foundation.

Curl your lashes and apply mascara.

Rub in cream blush to warm up cheeks.

## CLUMPY LASHES

Use a lash comb with metal teeth or a kid's soft toothbrush to coax the clumps out.

> Prevent clumped lashes by wiping off your mascara wand. The end should have almost no mascara on it.

## EXCESSIVE EYELINER

Remove the excess liner with a cotton swab.

Soften the look with a slightly lighter, but coordinating, eye shadow.

## CREASED EYE SHADOW

Pick up the excess by swiping a cotton swab over the crease.

Pat a little loose powder into it with your finger to absorb the shine.

## TOO MUCH BROW

Blend in overly applied brow pencil or powder with a cotton swab or sponge.

Dust on a small amount of translucent powder.

## OBVIOUS CONCEALER

Dab foundation over the concealer with your fingers. The warmth of your fingers will work the foundation into the skin and blend into the concealer.

Lightly pat a drop of moisturizer around the concealer to help blend the makeup colors where they meet.

## BLEEDING LIPSTICK

Wipe color toward the center of the mouth and then dab concealer on the surrounding skin.

Set with powder, applied with a cotton swab around the edges.

## LOUD LIP LINER

Obvious lip liner can be eliminated with concealer. Dip a brush into concealer and rub into the lip center.

## OVERLY BLUSHED

Blot the color off with a tissue. Separate the tissue and then press into the blush.

If this does not remove enough, take the other part of the tissue and dip it into powder and then press again.

## MESSY FOUNDATION

Smooth out cracks or cakey buildup by wetting a wash cloth and lightly going over the entire face. Even out the foundation and take away any moisture by blotting with a tissue.

# FAST FAKES

## BIGGER EYES

Dab a small amount of beige eye shadow on the center of your eyelids.

Apply on top of your regular eye shadow and then blend.

## MODEL CHEEKBONES

Apply bronze-colored blush underneath the cheekbone and along the jaw line.

Use a smaller contour brush rather than a fluffy blush brush.

Be sure to blend.

Finish with a light pink blush on the apples of the cheeks.

## FLAWLESS SKIN

Witch hazel immediately and temporarily shrinks pores by tightening the skin.

Apply to clean, dry skin with a cotton ball.

Follow up with makeup.

Trade face powder for bronzer. It will not only hide imperfections, it will make you look years younger. Apply over forehead, tops of cheeks, tip of nose, and chin.

## FULLER LIPS

Switch from matte to a shimmery gloss. Just apply it over your regular lipstick.

## INSTANT FACE LIFT

Gather hair into a ponytail at the crown.

Secure with an elastic band. Tease for fullness and smooth with a brush.

When you lift the hair, you give the illusion of lifting the face, too.

# HURRIED HAIR

## SPEEDY SHINE

Shine enhancers coat the hair cuticle to reflect light and make your hair look glossy. Always apply to damp hair for best results.

## QUICK **COLOR**

Color-depositing conditioners act as semi-permanent color in a pinch.

Coffee is perfect as a quick color refresher. Plus, the caffeine stimulates the scalp and increases circulation, resulting in more volume and body.

Make a pot of coffee and let it cool.

Shampoo, rinse, and then pour coffee on hair.

Leave on for ten minutes and then rinse.

# BODY MAGIC

## **THINNER**, SMOOTHER THIGHS

Shrink fat cells with coffee grounds.

Combine leftover warm coffee grounds with two teaspoons of sugar and a drop of vanilla extract. Apply over legs.

## **FIRMER** ARMS

Apply wet seaweed (available at health food stores) around upper arms.

With a rolling pin, roll over the area for a few minutes.

Remove and rinse with a vegetable brush.

## TEMPORARY **SLIMMER**

Add a cup of algae powder (available at health food stores) to bath water.

The algae reduces the water in fat cells, making you look slimmer.

Self tanner colors skin instantly. Use a formulation that allows you to see exactly where you're applying, which helps obtain the exact effect you want to have.

## APPETITE **SUPPRESSANT**

A cough drop containing menthol or eucalyptus stimulates your taste buds and sends a satisfaction signal to your brain, immediately ending your cravings.

## STAND UP **STRAIGHT**

Stand against a wall, pressing your body into it, elongating your body as if you're stretching it up along the wall.

Squeeze shoulder blades back so you're sticking your chest out.

Walk away from the wall and you'll look pounds thinner.

# FASHION FAKES

### **LENGTHEN** LEGS

Wear skirts with an asymmetrical hem to immediately give the illusion of longer, thinner legs.

Match your hose to your shoes.

### UPPER BODY

Wear ribbing to give arms a slimmer look.

A kimono-style top in satin will drape forgivingly over the tummy and flabby upper arms.

## A **BETTER** BEHIND

Ankle straps on shoes thin your lower legs while lifting your butt.

# Chapter 12

# AGE-DEFYING BREAKTHROUGHS

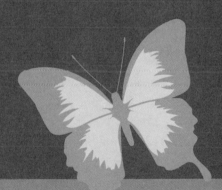

It's easier and faster than ever to fine tune your features and defy your age. It seems there are breakthroughs everywhere, and they're getting more and more refined. It's important to know the options that are out there and what's new in the world of keeping the years away.

## COSMETIC BREAKTHROUGHS

There are better-than-ever foundations and concealers with light-diffusing titanium dioxide and other minerals that create a smooth illusion and blend away imperfections by brightening.

## MICRODERMABRASION

Unlike dermabrasion, this technique won't leave skin reddened or scabby for days.

Remarkably, skin will be smooth and glowing immediately after the buffing.

In addition to removing old skin cells, the procedure encourages new cells to form and rejuvenates your complexion.

If you want to diminish fine lines, large pores, and acne scars, then this may be the procedure for you. You need a minimum of six sessions for the best effect and touch ups every one to two months depending on your skin and the result you want to achieve.

There's no recovery time, and you can even apply makeup immediately after the procedure.

## PHOTOFACIAL REJUVENATION

Used to get rid of complexion problems such as fine wrinkles, brown spots, red facial veins, large pores, facial hair, and rosacea.

## PULSED LIGHT

Used to deliver a precise amount of energy through the skin via a handpiece.

Usually done in five or six treatments.

Photo facials with pulsed light are good for women with rosacea.

## CO$_2$ LASER TREATMENTS

Used to vaporize deep wrinkles and scars without surgery.

A high-pulse laser light beam passes over skin and converts top superficial layers of skin into vapor. It feels like a bad sunburn, but the effects last about eight to ten years.

It can cost anywhere from one thousand to eight thousand dollars, depending on whether you're doing just part of the face or the entire face.

# BEYOND FACIALS

## GALVANIC CURRENT

Costs about one hundred dollars and uses ampoules of negative polarity, which are applied with a roller. This provides positive polarity into the deep layers of the skin. As the polarities balance against each other, the circulation of the skin is greatly maximized.

## OXYGENATING FACIAL

Costs anywhere from one hundred to two hundred dollars and is used to decongest the skin and restore balance. This procedure is excellent for oily skin.

## PANTY HOSE BREAKTHROUGHS

Even panty hose are getting into the fight against aging. You'll find companies have reinvented panty hose and are fighting to get their market share.

Check your lingerie department for:
- ❖ Anti-cellulite hose
- ❖ Moisturizing hose
- ❖ Non-slip panty hose that contains transparent silicone buttons that hold the heel in place.

# VARICOSE VEINS

## LASER THERAPY

This procedure can improve veins from 50 to 90 percent with a vasculight laser. This procedure can see complete closure of the blood vessels with just a few pulses.

## SCLEROTHERAPY

An irritating chemical solution is injected into varicose veins and it destroys them. This treatment forces blood to reroute to healthier veins.

## VASCULIGHT LASER

This laser treatment lets doctors create quick flashes of intense heat that seal large veins without sizzling the skin.

You spend thirty minutes or less in a doctor's office and the recovery is no more than wearing an Ace bandage for twenty-four hours.

Activity can be resumed after two days. Fifty to 80 percent of veins disappear after six weeks.

The cost is about two hundred to five hundred dollars per leg.

Make sure your doctor has had extensive experience using this laser.

## FACIAL ACUPUNCTURE

It's been used for more than three thousand years by the Chinese, and it is rapidly gaining popularity in other countries. Acupuncture is based on the belief that energy circulates throughout the body along well-defined pathways. Points on the skin along these pathways are linked to specific organs.

Sessions cost between fifty and seventy-five dollars.

## BOTOX

These popular injections involve the supervised use of the bacterium that causes botulism.

The injections block nerve impulses to muscles in the wrinkled area. The end result is a smooth outer area. Within twenty-four to forty-eight hours of treatment, wrinkles disappear for four to six months. Possible side effects include minimal bruising as well as rashes and swelling. There is also the possibility of temporary nerve damage. Plan on paying anywhere from four hundred to one thousand dollars per session.

## THERMA COOL

This is a radio-frequency device that combats early sagging and loss of radiance.

## MESOTHERAPY

This is a technique that was actually developed fifty years ago in Paris.

Mesotherapy is a series of up to five hundred tiny pricks during a thirty to sixty minute session that is said to liquefy fat anywhere on the body.

Expect to pay about two hundred and fifty dollars per session. Advocates claim that about 20 percent of patients lose a dress size or more after their first treatment. The majority lose a size after three sessions.

Ten sessions is the length of an average treatment.

## LIPOSUCTION FOR BREAST REDUCTION

Although liposuction has been around for a long time, nobody considered using it for breast reduction until recently. It's becoming increasingly popular now that they have.

It leaves no scars, requires only local painkiller, allows doctors to remove a lot more fat, and causes almost no bruising or swelling.

Most patients are back to work within two to three days with lighter, higher, and firmer breasts than they ever had before.

The costs should be covered by most insurance policies.

## DERMALOGEN

This is a filler used to plump up lips. It costs five hundred to seven hundred dollars a syringe plus two hundred dollars a year for storage fees.

# GETTING RID OF LEATHERY LAYERS

Amino fruit acid peels are the next generation of exfoliators. These acid peels differ from glycolic peels because they're less irritating. They're chemically buffered by amino molecules and improve skin tone, normalize skin cells, and boost collagen production. Most people have a series of six treatments, one a week.

# VEIN IMPLANTS

You've heard about collagen treatments where doctors plump up facial wrinkles.

Unfortunately, they wear off after about three or four months. Now there's a new procedure that uses varicose veins to wipe out facial lines. The doctor removes an unsightly varicose vein from the leg and then invisibly implants it beneath a facial wrinkle or laugh line.

The veins contain 70 percent pure collagen, so they supply the wrinkle with a continuous source of youth-enhancing collagen for about twenty years.

It takes about thirty minutes, leaves no scars, and costs between one thousand to two thousand dollars.

## CUTTING OUT CELLULITE

Don't you just wish you could take that hunk of cellulite and cut it off of your body?

Well, now you can, or at least you can have it done.

Subcision is a new type of cutting under the skin used to treat acne scars. Now it offers hope for cellulite.

The procedure is done under local anesthesia and involves breaking up cellulite with a sharp, knifelike needle. Some of the ligaments that attach the skin to the muscle below flatten pockets and smooth skin.

The patient can perform normally right after the procedure, but healing takes a month and requires wearing elastic tights to discourage bleeding under the skin and to prevent cellulite from reforming.

## VITAMIN K

The University of Miami School of Medicine did a study where they applied vitamin K to one side of the face and a placebo on the other twice daily after bruising. Vitamin K, they found, significantly reduced the severity of bruising.

Another study showed that vitamin K was highly effective in treating spider veins by dilating blood vessels.

## AGING TEETH BREAKTHROUGHS

Whiter teeth look younger. If your teeth are beginning to resemble old piano keys, then you may be looking older than you should. Years of coffee, cigarettes, and red wine have gone into the enamel, tinting your teeth darker. Consider cosmetic dentistry on your road to age defying.

## LASER WHITENING

A highly effective procedure that can be done in a dentist's office in an hour, laser whitening can whiten teeth dramatically and is well worth the investment of about five hundred to six hundred dollars.

## BONDING

A simple way to repair chips or close gaps between teeth. A clay-like material is sculpted onto a tooth. The price is between one hundred to two hundred dollars. Results last up to eight years. The downside to bonded teeth is that they stain easily.

## VENEERS

Thin porcelain barriers that offer better looking and straighter teeth. They are stain proof and can last up to fifteen years. The price is between seven hundred and nine hundred dollars a tooth.

In addition to giving you a younger smile, another benefit is that veneers can give you fuller lips. Dentists build out teeth about a quarter of an inch. This forces the lip to stretch out over the new line of the teeth and makes the lip look fuller.

## ASPIRIN

An Australian study had people taking low doses of aspirin (100 milligrams a day).

The aspirin takers had healthier gums than those who didn't. Aspirin protects ligaments that connect gums to teeth.

## PERIOSTAT

Dentists are now prescribing Periostat to patients after a deep cleaning treatment.

Taken for a few months, it restores gum health better than deep cleaning alone.

## PERIOCHIP

A tiny biodegradable chip is inserted around individual teeth, where it releases an antimicrobial.

# ANOTHER OPTION IS TO INJECT AN ANTIBIOTIC AROUND GUMS TO KILL HARMFUL BACTERIA.

# Chapter 13

# AGE-DEFYING SURGERY

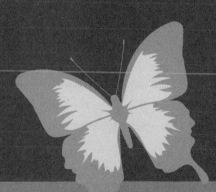

Everybody's doing it, from mothers to grandmothers to women in their thirties.

More and more women are choosing surgical alternatives to fighting age.

With strides that are being made in surgery today, the look has become much more natural looking. If plastic surgery is used to enhance your looks rather than try to make you a new person, it's just another spoke on the wheel of taking care of yourself.

Cosmetic procedures have come a long way from yesterday's windswept face lifts and ski slope nose jobs. If you are thinking about having "work" done, it's important to research the procedure you're seeking and to interview several surgeons who specialize in the field. Make sure that the surgeon is board certified. This way, you know that you're choosing a specialist who will have the proper credentials. Call the American Society of Plastic Surgeons to verify at 1-888-475-2784, or log on to www.plasticsurgery.org. Here you can get referrals and check doctors' credentials.

A reputable surgeon will provide you with photos and phone numbers of actual patients who have had the work that you're seeking. Always keep in mind that doctors only show pictures of their most successful work, and that photos can be retouched. Everybody is different, responds differently to surgery, and will have different results.

Surveys have been done gauging the effect of plastic surgery on women.

Women who have had plastic surgery in general live an average of ten years longer than their peers. Researchers feel that it's a boost in self image, creating greater optimism and a more youthful persona. It also creates more interest in the world and friendships.

# EYES

In their thirties and forties, women will most likely choose an eye lift as their first procedure. Ninety percent of the time, the eyes are the first to go.

Eye lifts have come a long way. Most surgeons now no longer cut large slices out of the upper lids and nothing from the lower lids of their patients because they have not developed enough sagging.

Most surgeons agree that if a woman has excess eyelid skin, she is a good candidate for an eye lift. If she has an eye that has fallen, giving the appearance of a droopy eye, then a brow lift would be helpful.

One way surgeons make the diagnosis is to feel the brow and see if it rests on or below the bone. Anything below would indicate a dropped brow.

An open brow lift, in which the surgeon makes an incision in the scalp from ear to ear to lift and tighten the skin, is the most aggressive brow lift.

## ENDOSCOPIC BROW LIFT

An endoscope is used to raise the brow, anchoring it to the skull with titanium tacks. It also requires a shorter recovery time and is less traumatic than an open brow lift. A woman in her thirties or forties requiring a brow lift would be the best candidate for this type of surgery since her tissues are still firm enough for this less-invasive approach.

# BREAST SURGERY

## BREAST AUGMENTATION

This is the insertion of an artificial implant that many aging women select to compensate for the loss of breast volume due to breastfeeding or weight fluctuations.

It takes three to five weeks until swelling goes down, and the final result will not be evident until several months later. Scars will almost always be visible

## BREAST REDUCTION

Oversized breasts can cause a variety of medical problems, which get worse with aging.

These include back pain, shoulder pain, headaches, and neck pain.

Breast reduction means tissue and skin is taken from the bottom of the breast and your nipple and areola are relocated but not detached.

Every year, surgeons are developing better techniques, and the movement is toward minimally invasive incisions.

Breast reduction is usually done in a hospital or outpatient clinic under general anesthesia. It is possible to be done under local anesthesia if fear of general anesthesia is holding you back.

This is one of the few cosmetic surgeries covered by most medical insurance companies.

## BREAST LIFT

A breast lift is the removal of excess breast skin to raise and recontour sagging breasts.

It takes two to three months until scars begin to fade. This is a permanent procedure unless there is significant weight gain followed by weight loss, which would cause breast tissue to expand and sag.

# TUMMY TUCKS AND LIPOSUCTION

## TUMMY TUCK

A tummy tuck is the removal of excess stomach tissue, with liposuction as a combined option, and the tightening of stomach muscles and removal of excess skin.

It takes two to three months until the support garment is no longer needed. Scars will be red and highly visible for several months.

## MINI TUMMY TUCK

Only a seven-inch incision right above the pubic hair line (leaving the belly button alone) makes this a less-invasive procedure. If you are looking to get rid of the middle to below-the-belt "pouch," perhaps the result of a pregnancy or two, then this is a realistic option.

You will be home the same day, but you should expect a small amount of pain because it is a deep incision. You should be back to normal after about two weeks.

You'll pay between four and five thousand dollars.

## LIPOSUCTION

The best candidate for liposuction is someone who is within 30 percent of their ideal body weight, has good skin elasticity, and whose skin hasn't wrinkled or begun to hang loose.

If you have fat deposits that have been resistant to diet and exercise, this is a great option that has been finessed through the years.

Liposuction is surgery, and with it comes soreness, bruising, skin sensitivity, numbness, and pain.

If you are considering liposuction, look for a board-certified plastic surgeon or skilled dermatologist. Ask around and get recommendations because the experience of the doctor will make all the difference with the results.

Ask the doctor what kind of liposuction will be done. There is conventional, tumescent, and ultrasonic.

Conventional liposuction uses a cannula, a long thin tube, to suck out fat.

With tumescent technique, the doctor injects a solution into the fatty tissue that anesthetizes the area. It causes the area to become firm and swollen (tumescent), which enables the surgeon to extract fat more accurately and uniformly, and thereby produces smoother results.

Ultrasonic liposuction uses sound waves to break up fatty deposits for speedy removal through larger incisions that often require stitches.

# FACE

## FACE LIFT

The best candidates for a face lift are those whose skin is still in good condition.

143

If you wait too long and the skin becomes thin, you won't get the optimal result.

Healing time is about a month, but with the right makeup you can go out in about two weeks.

## ENDOSCOPIC MID-FACE LIFT

This youth rejuvenator requires only four incisions, which include two inside the mouth and two behind the hairline, and a few stitches to ensure the tissue lift reestablishes high cheekbones and adds volume to the middle of the face. This creates an oval appearance.

This lift works best for women under fifty who don't have the severe sagging that would require a full face lift. It also is used as a touch up for an earlier face lift.

It's day surgery, but bruising and swelling can take up to five days to disappear. The average cost for an endoscopic mid-face lift is about four thousand dollars, as opposed the cost of a full face lift, which begins at around seven thousand dollars.

## CHEMICAL PEELS

Superficial laugh lines can be eliminated or greatly lightened with a chemical peel.

**Deep LAUGH LINES can be plumped up with natural fillers, such as fat.**

## CLOSED RHINOPLASTY

This is a less radical option for an aging and drooping nose. It is done with one or more incisions through the nostril. The surgery may also involve work on the inside lining, cartilage, and bone.

## LIP SCULPTURE

This procedure can improve an area's contours through surgical removal of fat cells.

It starts with a small incision, less than a quarter of an inch, through which fat is removed.

## LIP LIFT

The surgeon makes an incision along the line where the upper and lower lip meet. He removes a tiny amount of skin, then pulls the lip edge and stitches it in to its new position. Local anesthesia is usually sufficient. Your lips may be swollen and sore, and you'll want to apply a cold compress the first night.

The recovery is quick, and most people return to their regular activities within a day or two. It costs about one thousand dollars.

## MICROSUCTION

This is a form of liposuction and can be used to fix a slack jawline and horizontal neck creases. The doctor makes tiny holes under the chin or behind the ear lobes and, using a vacuum-like device, sucks fat from the corners of your mouth, jawline, chin, and neck.

Removing the fat will contour the lower face while the motion of cannula irritates the undersurface of the skin, stimulating it to tighten and look better.

# ARMS AND BUTTOCKS

## ARM LIFT

The surgeon makes an incision from your elbow to your armpit, removing the loose skin.

Then he tightens and sutures the remaining skin to the underlying tissue. If you have excess fat, it can be suctioned out at the same time.

The anesthesia is local with intravenous sedation. You'll be swollen and will need to restrict arm movement for about a week to prevent the sutures from opening.

This is the only surgical solution for sagging arms and you will have a long, visible scar.

## BATWING ARMS

Those arms that continue to wave goodbye long after you've stopped are the reason that many aging women won't show their arms. This is a difficult area to treat. If too much fat is suctioned out, then the sagging can be even worse.

Liposuction can make flabby arms thinner, but it cannot make flabby arms firm.

## BUTTOCKS LIFT

If your problem is excess skin on your buttocks and thighs, then a surgical lift is the procedure you should look into.

The surgeon makes an incision in the crease below the buttocks. In the case of a thigh lift, the incision is made in the crease of the groin area around the inside of the thighs and into the buttocks crease. If you're having your outer thighs done too, then the incision continues all the way around.

Excess skin is pulled tight, trimmed, and sutured to deep tissue. In the traditional thigh lift, the patient has to be moved several times, so it is a long surgery done under general anesthesia.

For three weeks you'll need to avoid putting pressure on the area to prevent tearing your sutures. Standing and lying down are permitted but no sitting.

## LASER SURGERY

The misconception is that laser surgery should be taken lightly. It's still surgery, but there are numerous procedures that can be done with lasers that formerly required much more extensive surgery.

Cosmetic laser surgery has many advantages over traditional surgery. It's quick and usually only needs a local anesthetic. Plus, it involves no incision and there's less recovery time. It can be used to erase everything from acne scars, birthmarks, and tattoos to varicose veins.

## CARBON DIOXIDE LASER RESURFACING

The purpose of this procedure is for skin to peel and heal more smoothly. Recovery takes about two weeks, with some pinkness for a few months that can easily be covered up with the right makeup.

## PHOTODERM/ PULSED-DYE LASER

This procedure fixes broken capillaries, red blotches, and red birthmarks. As tissue is lasered, the red mark or blood vessel is destroyed. It feels like a drop of hot wax on the skin. There is little risk of scarring in this procedure.

# Chapter 14

# REAL-LIFE AGE DEFYING

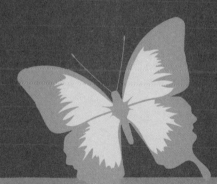

The questions I asked women while collecting stories for this chapter were general, yet personal.

1. What are you doing to fight aging?
2. Would you consider plastic surgery?
3. If you did have any surgery done, why did you do it? Do you regret it?
4. What rules have you broken?
5. How has your perception of yourself changed through the years?
6. What is your favorite age-defying trick?

Although each woman I interviewed related differently in her approach to aging, the common thread was an "A-ha!" moment. Even though outside intervention often played a part in their epiphanies, the sense of peace came from within.

# REAL-LIFE AGE-DEFYING BEAUTY TRICKS

## THE CASE FOR RHINOPLASTY

"My big, slightly crooked nose had a real impact on my behavior when I was younger. It gave me a loud personality. I realize now that the behavior was an attempt to take attention away from my nose. I'd continually wonder if people were thinking about my personality or my nose. It made me very self-conscious. Once I decided to change my nose I looked for a surgeon. Now I have confidence. I have a nose that is less than perfect, smaller, and I can go meet people being me. I wish I had done this years ago. I wear more makeup because I feel more attractive, and I'm outgoing without resorting to being loud."

—Celia, 48

"My nose seemed to have grown over the years, until it seemed it was almost touching my upper lip. It was sagging quicker than any other part of my body. Once I had my nose done, it picked up my entire face. I had actually thought I needed a face lift, but so far so good. I had gone to three surgeons and chose the one who recommended the least amount of surgery."

—Sharon, 47

## LASER RESURFACING

"When I reached my mid thirties, I became very self conscious about the scars on my face from acne. I had become used to them, but as my skin started to show signs of aging, I realized the scarring was getting worse. My skin was beginning to look very pitted, and the scars were starting to look like groove lines. I know my friends felt sorry for me.

It didn't interfere with my life, but I was always self-conscious about my face. I'd find myself staring at other women, wishing my skin could look like theirs. Then I heard about laser skin resurfacing. After looking into it, I decided this was the procedure that I would allow myself. My face was very red and swollen afterward, but I could see that it was noticeably smoother immediately. It took a month for my skin to calm down, and I did have occasional flushing from it. Now I'm a changed woman a year and a half later. I'm no longer preoccupied with how my skin looks, and I feel the same as everyone else. I used to walk past mirrors without looking at myself. Now I don't think twice about reapplying my lipstick or powdering my nose in public. Of course, my skin isn't perfect, but who has flawless skin? My skin looks the same as everyone else's. I no longer have the fine lines that I started developing in my thirties, and it has given me additional confidence to think that my skin looks smoother and younger. But most important is that it makes me feel comfortable in my own skin."

—Liz, 40

## STRENGTH TRAINING

"I started exercising to strengthen my immune system. I'm seventy-eight years old, and I've been able to triple my strength, according to my doctor. I feel wonderful!

—Miriam, 78

## WATER WARRIOR

"I've learned that drinking a lot of water makes a difference in the fine lines in my face, so I've made it a point to drink eight full glasses of water a day. My skin's texture visibly changes and becomes a lot more dewy. I carry water with me all day long. I freeze a couple of bottles and let them defrost through my day."

—Lorraine, 37

## COMMON-SENSE DIETING

"In my twenties and thirties, I would run a lot and eat only healthy foods. I thought I was in great condition, but all of a sudden my hair began to fall out and my weight plummeted due to my overactive thyroid. My doctor told me to stop exercising, and I gained twenty pounds. When my thyroid stabilized, I found that even after I went back to running I could not lose all the weight. But I also felt calm about it. I ate real food, didn't go crazy at the gym, and didn't feel guilty. I now live with my weight and think about doing something physical every day. I would love to be ten pounds thinner, but I also am glad to have my hair back and be at peace with myself."

—Suzanne, 43

## NEW ROUTINES

"I've found that when I started using glycolic and alpha hydroxy moisturizers, my blackheads and clogged pores disappeared."

—Candice, 38

## COSMETIC DENTISTRY

"Although my crooked smile was cute when I was younger, when I turned forty it really started to affect me, and I found myself not wanting to smile as often. I had spoken to some people who had gone through cosmetic dentistry, and I decided to take this route. The treatment was done in two stages, and I was surprised at how pain free I was. I had to wear temporary veneers for a week while my permanent ones were being made. After the treatment I felt a little strange because I talked a little bit differently, but almost immediately I kept asking myself why I had waited so long. People ask me why I look so different. I personally feel that I look ten years younger. And I can't stop smiling, which is even more youth enhancing."

—Melissa, 42

## CLOTHES SCALE

"I keep my old clothes in the back of my closet to serve as a barometer to the changes in my body. I'll try them on every now and then. If they don't fit right or feel comfortable, I just start to walk more and eat a little less."

—Mary, 54

## HAIR REVIVAL

"Even though I vowed I would age gracefully, my gray hair had to go. I turned it into a golden blonde with highlighting around the face and crown for depth. Then I had the hairstylist teach me how to use the latest frizz-control products, such as silkening serum. I also learned the correct way to blow my hair straight. I think (and others agree) that I look about fifteen years younger."

—Kim, 61

## BEAUTY AND BALANCE

"I'm fifty-one years old, and even though I want to look good for my age, I also have to have a balanced life. I have a great job and I have a great family life with my husband and children, and I've found my own comfort level. I have stopped wearing anything that makes me look costumed, and if my makeup is too bright, I tone it down."

—Jeanne, 51

"I've let go of a lot of unrealistic expectations, and I've stopped comparing myself with actors or models. Instead, I've started comparing myself with real women, like my friends and relatives. It not only is more realistic, but it makes me feel a lot better about myself."

—Helen, 46

"I think of my look as a total package. I know that I need to give my body enough sleep, I need to exercise, and I need time to unwind. I've learned to tune in to my body and accept that I need intellectual challenges as well as physical challenges."

—Susan, 50

"I've learned not to look back and not to get stuck in an image that dates me. I'm always experimenting and I'm continually reassessing my hairstyle, hair color, and makeup as my hair and skin change. I've found that this is the easiest way to keep updating my look without having to spend a fortune on plastic surgery."

—Patricia, 45

"I've started breaking bad habits for good. I no longer do sunbathing, I've finally stopped smoking, I make sure I floss, and I've sworn off any fad diets. Basically, I've sworn off anything self destructive that I did in my twenties and thirties, and I feel a lot better."

—Tina, 43

## YOUTHFUL HAIR

"I've lost the frizz. I found that overpermed hair is not youthful, so I get a light body wave about four times a year."

—Flo, 66

## A SOFTER TOUCH

"I've switched to brown liner. I used to be the queen of black but have found it too harsh lately. I use a brown liquid liner on the upper lid only and a light brown shadow under my lower lashes to take attention away from crow's feet."

—Liz, 49

## GETTING REAL

"I've found that taking care of myself and doing what I need to do to stay current is important. I've also found that trying to turn back the clock is next to impossible. Anyone who overdoes it looks transparent to me as well as uncomfortable in their skin."

—Lana, 39

## LIVE WITH IT

"I have been blessed with certain features, which I play up. The ones I've fought with all my life I keep in the background with concealing techniques."

—Janet, 53

## BREAKING RULES

"I've felt more beautiful since I've started to live my life according to what gives me pleasure as opposed to what I should do. Little pleasures like baths, pedicures, yoga, dance, long walks (without speed walking), and relating to other people makes me feel younger than any cosmetic."

—Veronica, 52

## GETTING BACK TO BASICS

"I cook a lot from scratch and that makes me feel connected to the earth. I've also transformed a few of my chemical concoctions into natural treatments using avocados, cucumbers, and strawberries. I feel that the same satisfaction I get from cooking I also get in my beauty routines."

—Daisy, 36

## GET A LEG UP

"Even though I've become a bit heavier as I age, I don't hesitate to show off my still-shapely legs. It makes me feel great and takes the attention to my good spot."

—Karen, 55

## DEFEND AND PROTECT

"I've found that I need more foundation and concealer to even out my complexion. I also make sure it has sunscreen in it so that I can be protected from further damage."

—Carmela, 59

## DON'T SWEAT THE SMALL STUFF

"To me there's a positive side to aging, and that is as I get older I no longer seek approval for what I do. I'm no longer easily embarrassed and it's a liberating, powerful feeling.

The confidence I now have shines right through my skin. Little things just don't bother me anymore."

—Maria, 47

## SKIN CHANGES

"When I reached sixty years old, I decided to stop aging with an aggressive skin care regime. I wash my skin with Evian water and wear sunblock and hats when I go outside. I even wear sunblock on my hands."

—Evelyn, 68

"I remember that my mother often said if you don't want wrinkles on your brow, then be careful not to crease it. I stopped frowning from that day on."

—Mary, 58

"I have a full-body massage twice a week. Not only does it relax me and invigorate my skin, it makes me more body aware."

—Gina, 61

## SELF EDUCATION

"I was a strict vegetarian. But as a vegetarian I was eliminating so many foods that I was getting weak. This forced me to learn a lot about nutrition. Now I'm the healthiest I've been in my life, and I don't get all the colds and viruses I used to. Another plus is that my skin and hair have never looked better."

—Megan, 42

## NO MORE CRAZY COLORS

"I've finally come to the decision that I look a lot better in earthy colors than cosmetics that never possibly came from nature."

—Chris, 55

## INSIDE OUT

"After years of smoking, I love the feeling that comes after a workout. Granted, I'll never become a marathon runner, but I have come to love the feeling of being spent, of being cleansed, and it's the best beauty treatment I can give myself."

—Gina, 41

## SELF KINDNESS

"As I'm aging, I've learned not to drive my body like a machine. If I do, it rebels on me.

I've learned to key into its displeasure, and now I pamper myself as much as I push myself."

—Brenda, 53

## FAMILY TIES

"Most of my family is obese, so diet and exercise is very important to me. I have to weigh myself each morning since it can so easily get away from me. When I come back from a family event, I know that I need to cut back for the next few days. There are still triggers from my childhood that I can't avoid, so I've learned to live with them as they are."

—Carol, 44

## ONE AT A TIME

"I am trying to repair years of sun damage, so I've begun to use acids. I've found that some of the lines have become less apparent. I haven't had plastic surgery yet, but when I can't perform self repair, or the cost of the products I'm using becomes too high, it's definitely in the running."

—Lucille, 49

## DOMINO EFFECT

"Two years ago I treated myself to a face lift, and it has helped me put things into the right order. Now that I like what I see in the mirror, it urges me on to keep up with the rest."

—Lana, 56

## LIGHTENING UP

"I had breast reduction surgery five years ago for cosmetic reasons and because they were so heavy. My back was constantly hurting. Finally I feel freer, and I think the scars were more than worth it. People either didn't notice or thought that I had lost weight. Now I feel more proportioned."

—Alana, 42

## TAKING OFF THE LAYERS

"I got a mild chemical peel, and I found that it really does make a difference in my complexion and makes me more confident to go out without makeup."

—Karen, 49

## TAKING IT BACK

"After I turned sixty, I finally started doing things for myself. My children were grown and I decided to take myself off the shelf. I've allowed myself some surgery. I've had a face lift and liposuction and it's helped so much with accepting the whole aging process."

—Linda, 64

## CLEANING OUT

"I had endermologie to clean out my lymphatic system. It uses rollers to facilitate circulation and it is supposed to eliminate toxins and cellulite deposits. I now feel that I have much better tone."

—Sally, 45

## LOOKING GOOD

"I had lasik surgery to correct my eyesight permanently. My eyes got very dry with contact lenses, and it has helped enormously. I was very nervous, but the difference it has made for me has been tremendous. I'm having so much fun experimenting with eye makeup that I could never wear before."

—Ginger, 48

## JUST ENOUGH

"I decided to have a mid-face lift to get a better jawline. It made me less nervous than if I was having a full face lift and it made a remarkable difference."

—Cara, 51

"I had an eyebrow lift. People kept telling me that I didn't need it, but when I got to the point of looking in the mirror and not recognizing myself, I went for it. I'm so glad I did. I no longer look constantly tired. The person you need to listen to is yourself."

—Ellen, 54

## FIND YOUR OWN GROOVE

"I found that doing exercises that I like causes me to keep doing them. I thought I hated exercising, but I just hated certain exercises."

—Danielle, 32

"I go into the backyard and jump rope. It's cheap, quick, and it brings me down memory lane."

—Megan, 36

## WORTH EVERY PENNY

"I had veneers done, which cover the front of the tooth, unlike caps, which cover the entire tooth. People who knew me thought I looked great. Yes, it was a lot of money, but only after getting them did I realize how my teeth had worn down and yellowed over the years."

—Denise, 52

"The only thing that was bothering me was the number 'eleven' sitting between my brows. Those two pesky lines made me look like I was constantly frowning. So every five months I treat myself to Botox injections. It's something that I am glad to trade in my daily lattes for."

—Kathy, 46

## LIP TRICKS

"I am trying to get my lips to look more pouty without getting collagen shots. I've used peppermint oil and cinnamon oil mixed in with my lipstick. It's not permanent, but it's a lot cheaper."

—Jane, 31

## MAKEUP MANEUVERS

"Switching from a dark lipstick with lip liner to a soft and more transparent lip gloss is not only easier to wear, it takes attention away from my thinning lips."

—Jane, 58

"I found myself overcompensating for my fading hair color and pallor by wearing a lot of face makeup. It didn't look natural and made me look like I was wearing a mask.

I brightened my hair and stopped wearing powdered products and found that I looked a lot younger."

—Rachel, 62

"No one dared to tell me that my very dark eyebrows were no longer matching my hair and were giving me a weird look. It took some vacation pictures for me to see the evidence. They were also too heavy. First I had them lightened and then had them professionally waxed. The result was amazing. My features softened, and it gave me a more refreshed look."

—Willie, 46

"I cried, but I knew it was time to update my cosmetic bag. Out went the powdery shadows in colors that I never wore like green, yellow, purple, and orange. Most I had been gifted with when I made another cosmetic purchase, and well, I just couldn't bear to throw them out. I also threw out all my bright-colored blushes which, rather than flattering, looked clownish. I don't know why I kept them, but not having them anymore urged me to look for the right stuff!"

—Sandy, 49

"Too many colors on my face made me take too much time putting on my makeup before heading out the door every morning. It was impossible to coordinate colors in less than thirty minutes. I also had the sense that all the trouble I went to didn't make me look any better. A friend suggested that my makeup made me look theatrical. Now I stay with one color scheme. It saves me time, and I get lots of compliments."

—Gia, 35

"My friends would ask me where I was going when I wasn't even dressed up! It finally dawned on me that was wearing the wrong kind of makeup. I found that it was my mirror that was doing me in. Doing my makeup by natural light turned out to be what I needed."

—Talia, 31

"I give my eyes an instant lift by using eye shadow only at the outer corners and creating a little upturn at the ends, heading toward the outside of my eyebrows."

—Mary Ellen, 37

"I carry wet chamomile tea bags with me during the day to refresh my face. Usually two teabags in a sandwich bag will take me through the entire day."

—Kendra, 50

"To keep my lipstick from bleeding, I seal it in by patting a matching color blush over it after blotting."

—Patti, 45

"My favorite way to disguise the lines around my eyes is to apply a small amount of eye shadow under the outer corner of my lower lashes. I make sure to connect it to the upper corner and always use a dark color so the attention goes to the shadow and not my crow's feet."

—Amanda, 44

"I always make sure that my eyebrows are the emphasis of my face. I find that they bring attention away from the sags and bags on the rest of my face."

—Chynna, 67

"My favorite age-defying trick is to take a little bit of my blush and pat it on my eyelids over my shadow. It brightens my eyes."

—Cilla, 39

"I take a very small amount of loose powder and press it into the inner corners of my eyes with my fingers. It takes away the darkness from that area and also prevents any eye shadow from seeping into the area."

—Pam, 54

"I prefer to blot my foundation on with my fingers. It looks younger because the warmth of my fingers makes it easier to blend and provides a dewy finish."

—Donna, 48

"As a woman of color, I have a hard time finding the perfect color foundation. The solution for me is two-way foundation. I can use it wet in the morning and touch up dry during the day."

—Sheila, 55

# AGE DEFYING WITH STYLE

## ACCESSORIZING

"I love wearing belts but find that as I get older my waist line is getting thicker. I've found that allowing the belt to sit slightly lower on my waist (almost to my hips) gives me the illusion of a smaller waist without binding."

—Frieda, 46

"More than two pieces of jewelry makes me look as if I'm trying too hard. I find that a pared-down look is not only more slimming, but more chic."

—Beverly, 63

## MONOCHROMATIC STYLING

"Staying with the same color line has really helped pare down my wardrobe and looks more pulled together."

—Jenny, 59

## TEXTURED HOSE

"A slight opaque texture hides my leg veins and makes my legs look slimmer, especially when I match my skirt and shoes with them."

—Carol, 53

## FABRICS

"As I age, I have found that I look much better in higher-quality fabrics. They drape my body in a more forgiving way."

—Shauna, 57

## COLOR COORDINATION

"Loud prints and big patterns are impossible to wear, and although they can look really fun on young beach kids, after thirty-five I found that they no longer looked cute. I always choose sophistication over fun fabrics when I'm on a limited budget. The only exception that I make is when I'm vacationing at a resort. Then I go for a big-printed pair of slacks (usually tropical). I subdue the pants by choosing the rest of my outfit based on the background color of the print."

—Samantha, 66

## SHOE SENSE

"There is something I notice that really ages a woman's look. It's run-down shoes. I keep mine in top condition or I throw them away. I find that not only do I look a lot more polished, but I have more support so I walk better."

—Diane, 54

"My motto is never to wear anything tied unless it's a sneaker. I know there's lots of fun styles out there, but tied shoes look orthopedic on me now that I'm no longer twenty."

—Coleen, 48

"Wedged shoes allow me to get a higher heel without killing myself when I'm dashing around all day. There are great styles out there, and most wedged shoes also usually have a non-slip sole."

—Elizabeth, 34

# Chapter 15

# AGE-DEFYING EXTREMES

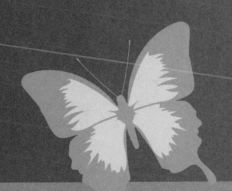

Oh, the things that have been done in pursuit of beauty!

From the reckless:

"I was desperate to put volume in my thinning, aging hair. I thought, hmm, Miracle Gro works to accelerate plant growth, maybe it will help grow some hair. I ended up with a terribly burned scalp instead."

—Carly, 56

To the ridiculous:

## APPETITE SUPPRESSING EYEGLASSES

More than one woman in my focus group has used these in a desperate attempt to lose weight. These colored lenses are supposed to project an image to the retina that lessens the desire to eat. The women claimed that it didn't help, and the FDA states that there is no evidence to support the claims behind it.

## SLIMMING SOAP

The company that makes this seaweed soap alleges that the *Wall Street Journal* endorsed its usage. In reality, the article was less than favorable. It quoted a medical anthropologist who claimed that there was no link between seaweed and weight loss. Another quote from a medically trained herbalist quipped that eating the soap would be more effective than bathing with it.

## WEIGHT-LOSS SLIPPERS

Sold on the internet and reported to be very popular in Japan, these slippers are made deliberately too short so that the heel of the foot hangs over the edge. The slippers are supposed to be a cross between reflexology and magnet therapy. There's a bulging cinder that applies pressure to the arches while magnets located in the slippers supposedly stimulate the nerve endings of the soles. The claim is that the slippers will increase your metabolism naturally. The FDA says there is no evidence that the slippers work.

## HORSE URINE

Celebrities started it, and now cultists are actually being injected with it in an attempt to increase metabolism.

# WHAT IS EXTREME?

## FACE

Lifted, masked, peeled, toned, massaged, moisturized, covered with foundation, highlighted, shaded, contoured, and blushed.

## EARS

Pierced, pinned back and lobes lifted, and reduced.

## BROWS

Tweezed, waxed, penciled, tattooed, and dyed.

## LASHES

Dyed, curled, and dressed with mascara.

## LIDS

Lined, shadowed, and surgically altered.

## LIPS

Glossed, frosted, and "plumped" with collagen.

## NOSE

Implanted, reduced, turned up or turned down.

## HAIR

Permed, straightened, teased, rinsed, tipped, streaked, chunked, dyed, curled, sprayed, moussed, and gelled.

## TEETH

Capped, veneered, whitened, and even removed to accent cheekbones.

## NAILS

Manicured, polished, painted, covered, and falsified.

## BODY HAIR

Removed by electrolysis, depilatories, waxing, tweezing, shaving, lasering of the upper lip, chin, brows, underarms, legs, and bikini line.

## BREASTS

Augmented with implants, reduced, lifted, and padded.

## BUTTOCKS

Plumped, lifted, and reduced.

## STOMACH

Stapled (to reduce food intake), tucked surgically, and surgically liposuctioned.

## HIPS, THIGHS

Firmed and reduced (with machines or surgically), dissolution of cellulite.

## FEET

Reshaped by high-heeled, pointed shoes, toes amputated to fit into these shoes.

There seems no limit nowadays to the extent that women (and men) are prepared to go to in order to look younger, thinner, and more attractive.

Forget false eyelashes and wigs, we are now talking scalpels, implants, and liposuction!

Cosmetic surgery among top celebrities has been commonplace for quite some time now, but these days, we wouldn't be too hard pressed to find ordinary women on the street who are more plastic than real! Indeed, in some circles, having multiple face lifts has become a status symbol: the more you have, the higher you are in the rankings.

Cher is reputed to have spent a million dollars on having herself lifted, pinned, shaped, tucked, contoured, and implanted so that she would look just like a million dollars!

Demi Moore is over forty and still looks fabulous. The tabloids claim she has spent around $380,000 on cosmetic surgery. The *London Daily Mail* claims she has had an operation to reduce her breast implants; liposuction on her stomach, buttocks, and thighs; collagen for her lips; and porcelain veneers for her teeth.

## EXTREME MODELING

Some girls, in a desperate attempt to alter their bodies in order to enter or remain competitive in the modeling industry, have gone so far that they have permanently become disabled or disfigured. The unrealistic standard of the modeling industry is the ultimate example of beauty gone overboard. I've been in the industry since the age of thirteen, and after forty years behind the runways, I am still amazed at how much abuse these girls are willing to inflict on their own bodies.

## TOILET PAPER

I have seen models make spitballs out of small pieces of toilet paper and actually swallow them with large glasses of water in an effort to assuage their appetites. Somehow they've convinced themselves it is the ultimate fiber.

## LAXATIVES

When I was a model, there was a notoriously cold agent who would routinely pass out laxatives the night before a big shoot or runway show so that the models would have absolutely flat tummies for the clients.

## REMOVING BONES

I've interviewed dozens of surgeons, and not one will admit that this is acceptable or was ever done. I've seen suspicious marks. In the late fifties and early sixties, before liposuction, there were runway models who spoke openly about having ribs removed.

## TEETH WHITENING

Veneers are now almost a necessity in the industry. But there are models just starting out who have no money and no sense. A dentist allegedly told one of them (and unfortunately bad advice travels too fast in the modeling world) that it was safe to whiten their teeth with scrubbing cleanser like Comet or Ajax. It is not safe. It wears off your enamel and it's toxic. It was created to clean tubs, not teeth. Don't do it, and don't even think about it. There are whiteners out there that have become fast and inexpensive.

At a photo shoot I found a model who had applied Liquid Paper to her teeth in an attempt to disguise the stains.

## DIETING

Days of not eating, bingeing and purging, chewing but not swallowing. Not only have I seen this in the modeling world, but with the "ladies who lunch." Severe dieting has entered the mainstream, and it sets up a life threatening cycle. I'm seeing more and more of these dangerous routines in aging women.

## DRUGS

I'm not even going to go into the dangerous drugs. Any drug can become a danger when it's abused, especially an appetite suppressant. More than one model has fainted or fallen off the runway because of the "one is effective, three is what I need to really control my appetite" mentality.

Here's Lisa, who struggled for years to stay in the modeling world at five feet nine, 115 pounds:

"When I entered modeling at the age of sixteen, I was a healthy 140 pounds. This was my natural, athletic weight (I ran track). My agency made me immediately lose twenty pounds. Even though this weight was light for me, I could live with it if I watched everything I ate. Then the waif movement took over, and I wasn't getting as many jobs.

The only way I was able to get down to 115 pounds was to crash at the end of my day of eating a few bites of salad and a slice or two of turkey. I would take a Xanax and a glass of wine and watch tapes of runway shows. I finally took myself out of the loop when it took all my energy to maintain that weight. I'm now a comfortable 145 pounds and I think I look better than ever."

—Lisa, 42

# Chapter 16

# AGE-DEFYING PROBLEMS/SOLUTIONS

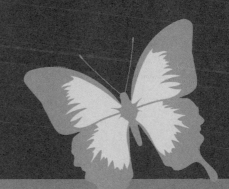

I can't tell you how many questions I get in a single day. It doesn't matter whether it's by email, phone, a lecture, or a photo shoot. There are the questions that come up consistently, and here they are. I hope that you'll refer to this section when you don't have time to track me down.

Dear Diane:

I am a woman of color with oily skin. Is there a gel blush that blends into colored skin and looks natural? I understand that creams don't work well with oily skin.

—Beverly

Dear Beverly:

I would suggest that you use a cream blush that turns to powder when it is applied. Powdered blush on top of oily skin just sits there and looks unnatural. If you prefer to use a gel blush, and they do complement the skin more naturally, then dip your finger into loose blush powder and mix with a small amount of gel. Don't try to apply gel blush to already powdered skin. All you'll get are unflattering streaks.

Dear Diane:

I've been purchasing a face cream containing pro-retinol. It is supposed to help with face and neck firming. Do these products really work and are they safe to use?

—Janet

Dear Janet:

That product is fine for wrinkle reducing, but if you're looking for firming results, then you need to look for these three ingredients, not necessarily in this order: wheat protein, copper, and grape seed oil. There are a variety of these products in different price categories. If you can find the ingredients, there is no need to pay a lot.

Dear Diane:
I have a light blue makeup base/color corrector, but I'm not sure how to use it. Every time I use it, I end up looking too pale or slightly ashy. Do I sheer it down with my moisturizer or mix it with my foundation? What are my alternatives, as I really don't want to toss it?
—Susan

Dear Susan:
Actually, makeup artists create their own color correctors by mixing blue eye shadow with concealer or foundation to correct ruddy tones and broken capillaries. By mixing our own, they are able to exact the color.

Since you don't want to toss this product, my suggestion is that you apply it before your foundation and allow it to set. If you still aren't getting the desired outcome, then try adding a little blue eye shadow to it. If it looks blue when you apply it, you've used too much. Here's another hint: add yellow eye shadow to concealer or foundation and apply to under eye circles. It color corrects dark undertones.

Dear Diane:
For the past two years, I've been getting this terrible rash around my eyes when I wear makeup, especially near the outer corners. The dermatologist diagnosed dermatitis and said to apply hydrocortisone when I get a breakout. But the cortisone makes the area by my eyes dry and wrinkly. What can I do?
—Brenda

Dear Brenda:
I checked with my own dermatologist on this, and she agrees that hydrocortisone is too strong to be used around the eye area by itself. The suggestion is to mix it with a small amount of vitamin E. Just break open the capsule of vitamin E and add it to a small application of

hydrocortisone. Then gently tap it onto the eye area.

As for your makeup and adequate coverage, I recommend that you apply a two-way foundation that goes on wet but dries to a powder. This will be more forgiving to the skin and will dry to a protective finish. Plus, you can apply it dry throughout the day so that any redness that reappears can be quickly and adequately covered so that you can enjoy more confidence.

Dear Diane:
How do you buy a bra that truly fits right? I am a 42C—at least that is what I usually buy. However, I just can't seem to find a bra that supports me and makes me look good.
—Lori

Dear Lori:
You're not alone. Eight out of ten women are wearing the wrong bra size (usually too small!).

This is because we don't know how to measure our breasts, and we're too modest to ask an expert.

It not only affects the way our clothes look and feel, but wearing inadequate support can cause breasts to sag and age prematurely. First, measure your band size. While wearing a bra, pull a tape measure around your torso above the breasts and add one inch. Round up if you get an odd number like 35.

Dear Diane:
I often fall asleep before removing my makeup at night. What are the consequences of this?
—M.H.

Dear M.H.:
Of course, we are all guilty of that occasional lapse. But it's not good for your skin. While you're sleeping, your skin needs to "breathe" in order to restore and renew cells.

Evening is also when beauty treatments do their best work. At the very least, remove your face makeup. Leaving a bit of mascara or lipstick is not a good idea, but not as damaging. Now, if you do forget to take off your face makeup, do not use soap the next day. Instead, use a gentle cold cream or other non-irritating remover.

Dear Diane:
Although I have a fair complexion, my under-arms and inner thighs are very dark. How can I get rid of this?

—Joyce

Dear Joyce:
Simply take a little baking soda and mix it with enough lemon juice to make an easily spread-able exfoliant/paste. Rub it into the area and allow it to set for about a minute. Follow up with a fading cream that contains 2 percent hydroquinone. Use this overnight as if it were a regular moisturizer.

Dear Diane:
I have been through almost every foundation known to woman and I can't seem to find one that lasts all day without coming off or leaving a nasty yellow/orange tint to my skin. Can you help me?

—Dutchess

Dear Dutchess:
The method I use on my models and celebrities to keep their foundation from melting under hot lights will ensure all-day coverage without the mess for you. Prime your skin with only the smallest amount of moisturizer to allow even coverage of the foundation. If you have extremely oily skin, you can skip this step entirely. Next, switch to a wet/dry (usually called

two-way) foundation. You can use it slightly wet with a sponge or apply it dry. This type of foundation is not only long lasting, but blends in with most skin types for a natural look without the unflattering tint. Plus, it can easily be retouched by wrapping the sponge with a small amount of foundation and gently blotting.

Dear Diane:

I've noticed that some of my fragrance-laced lotions tend to get runny and watery if I don't use them in a timely manner. Is there anything that can be added to these lotions to turn them back into their original consistency (i.e., cornstarch or something like it)?

—Kristina

Dear Kristina:

Check the expiration date. Unless they are old, chances are that the contents have settled. You'll need to mix it with a straw or a skewer stick, since merely shaking it won't move the bottom, where the settling has occurred. If, however, there is any strange odor or color to the lotion, then you should throw it away.

Dear Diane:

Please tell me what to do about uneven skin tones. This is a problem for me. Tanning isn't an option. Do you have any suggestions as to what I should do?

—Wendy

Dear Wendy:

Since you don't want to look tan, a tinted moisturizer is not for you. It wouldn't give you enough coverage. You need to match foundation to the color of your jawline. This will give you the base color of your skin. Before you apply your foundation, you can correct your uneven color with concealer. A small dab goes a long way. Use a color that is as close to your jawline as possible. Using a concealer that is too light gives off a ghostly glow. A concealer that is too dark casts unflattering shadows. The foundation that blends easiest (and is also the most forgiving) is a two-way foundation (wet/dry). This can blend over the concealer without erasing it.

Dear Diane:

I sit behind a computer all day. I get so busy that I sometimes spend more than seven hours just sitting and replying to emails and phone calls. What's a good exercise for me to do at my desk?

—Elizabeth

Dear Elizabeth:

Your dilemma is shared by many of us. First, be sure to get up and walk around at least once an hour, even if it's just to the door to get a bit of fresh air. This will help circulation and ease back pain. Keep a couple of one-liter soda bottles at your desk to work your arms.

While you're downloading, grip your chair and use your arms to lift your body slightly off your seat and hold for ten to fifteen seconds. You can also do heel raises to work your calves, overhead stretches, and isometrics like holding your tummy in to the count of twenty. Don't forget the buttocks squeeze, another big fighter of "chair spread." Squeeze your buttocks to the count of thirty. There are lots more, but these are my favorites.

Dear Diane:

I am sixty-four years young. What exercise if any is good for the underarm? I'm talking about the area from the shoulder to the elbow.

—Kaye

Dear Kaye:

Oh, you mean that area of your arms that continues to wave goodbye long after you've stopped! Work that spot by placing the palm of your hand flat on a steady chair. Holding a small weight like a one-liter bottle of soda or a can of soup in your other hand, lean over and bring your arm back as far as you can. Hold for five seconds. Repeat ten times and then switch sides. As you become stronger, you can fill the soda bottle with sand or salt.

Dear Diane:
What is the best over-the-counter wrinkle reducer?

—Mary

Dear Mary:
The most effective way to combat wrinkling is actually nature's way. Vitamin C helps prevent and minimize wrinkles by boosting collagen, which holds skin in place. There are many creams on the market featuring vitamin C. To save money, head to the drugstore and purchase ester C powder. Add a small amount to your cleanser for a super-powered exfoliant and wrinkle reducer. Follow up by adding a capsule of vitamin A to any basic moisturizer. Using these products as "add ins" gives the product more potency as well as dollar savings.

Dear Diane:
I am a forty-year-old female, and I have a few white hairs growing on my chin. Is plucking them with tweezers the best way to remove them?

—Judy

Dear Judy:
Since you have just a few white hairs, tweezing them will keep them in check. To make the process less painful, apply a bit of Anbesol (yes, the toothache remedy) before tweezing.

Dear Diane:

I am a forty-five-year-old woman who enjoys skiing with my family and friends. Unfortunately, my skin is very sensitive to the cold and wind. What is a good product I can put on my face to avoid windburn?

—Paula

Dear Paula:

Professional skiers use bag balm (also called udder balm) to protect their faces. You can find it at most drugstores or mass merchandisers. It was originally used to prevent cow udders from chafing in milking machines. The secret is out: it works wonderfully! Remember to always apply it over clean skin.

Dear Diane:

At age sixty-two, I would like to know what modifications I need to make in my eye makeup. How much is enough? How much is too much? I have always used makeup, and my eyes have always been my best feature.

—Rosa-Lee

Dear Rosa-Lee:

Good for you for knowing to play up your best feature. A few changes are in order. The first consideration is to switch to neutral colors on the eyelid. Then bring definition to the eye with a soft pencil. A hard pencil or liquid liner would look too harsh.

My trick is to both seal in the pencil and soften the look by applying a matching shadow over the line. Apply a slightly darker shadow on the outside of the eye in an upward "V" shape. The point of the "V" should be directed to the outside brow. Don't forget to curl your lashes to provide even more definition. Use a soft pencil to fill in your brows. And don't forget, mascara is the finishing touch.

Dear Diane:

I have noticed lately that my eyelashes have become brittle and broken off. It seems to be taking a long time for them to grow back. I actually have a bald spot from my missing eyelashes. What can I do to help them grow back faster?

—Diana

Dear Diana:

A lot of lash breakage is a result of incorrect usage of one of my favorite tools: the lash curler. Here's the correct way to curl. Clamp your curler at the base of your lashes, and then gently "walk" it out to the tip. Be sure to clamp down (not too hard!) along the way.

Also be sure to always look for a mascara that is combined with a conditioner. You'll be able to coat your lashes while nourishing them. No more brittle lashes that fall out. While they do grow out, disguise the "bald spots" by drawing along the lash line with liquid liner.

Dear Diane:

What is the best way to cover gray roots for blonde hair in between professional color foils?

—Kerry

Dear Kerry:

Here's what we do in the industry. Purchase yellow sidewalk chalk and apply it to the roots with a shadow brush. It will wash out when you shampoo! This is a big beauty secret of TV anchors!

Dear Diane:

I do not have a few little facial hairs. I have a rough, coarse BEARD! I've tried depilatory creams and other things, yet nothing seems to work. I really can't afford the expense, time, or pain of electrolysis. Do you have any suggestions?

—Manly-in-the-morning

Dear Manly-in-the-morning:
Your easiest solution may be to shave your face. It's an old wives' tale that your hair will grow back heavier. Face shaving has been an insider secret for years in the modeling industry. It allows makeup to go on smoothly and flawlessly. As a bonus, occasional face shaving is an effective exfoliator. Use a razor made for sensitive skin.

Dear Diane:
I've heard you can use an egg for two different types of facials. The egg white for one, and the yolk for another. Would you please explain the difference between the two treatments?
—Leslie

Dear Leslie:
The egg white is an oil-absorbing mask, and can also be used as a temporary face lift. The egg yolk is a rejuvenating treatment. Both should be applied all over the skin and allowed to dry before removing. The egg white can actually be used as a firmer under your makeup.

Dear Diane:
When I walk for thirty minutes or longer, my legs start itching. What can be the cause of this and what I can do to lessen this factor?
—Marissa

Dear Marissa:
You can help prevent friction by applying cornstarch to your thighs before beginning your walk. It will help absorb the perspiration that is most likely causing the itching. Cornstarch is an anti-chafing, extremely absorbent powder.

Dear Diane:

I have a constant dark line on my upper lip. I have tried many things—even face bleach—to lighten it, yet it still persists. How do I get rid of it?

—Anonymous

Dear Anonymous:

Purchase ester C in powder form (available at health food stores) and mix it with enough lemon juice to make a paste. Apply it to the upper lip area with your finger, allow it to set for a moment, and then rinse off. Follow up by patting on the contents of a vitamin E capsule as a follow up.

Dear Diane:

Do you have suggestions on how to maintain fresh breath, even if it involves changing eating habits? It's embarrassing to have bad breath. I brush in the morning, but after a while my breath goes back to morning breath.

—S.V.

Dear S.V.:

First, check with your dentist and physician. Barring any health problems, there are remedies to ensure sweeter breath. When brushing your teeth, don't forget to brush your tongue. Make it a part of your regimen. Also note that dentists recommend that you brush your teeth for at least two minutes. Finally, chew a few fennel seeds. Fennel is rich in an antiseptic that destroys bacteria.

Dear Diane:

I have hyperhidrosis (excessive sweating of the hands, face, and other areas). A lot of it is mainly in my underarms, and I can't take it anymore, especially in this heat. It's also a problem for me in the middle of winter. Please help!

—Melina

Dear Melina:

Your condition is now being treated by some physicians with Botox shots. The shots virtually stop perspiration for up to four months. If your physician doesn't recommend this procedure (it is repetitive and costly), there are a select few antiperspirants that truly stop the sweating. Mitchum has one that models use, but there are other brands. After applying antiperspirant, allow it to dry and pour a small amount of cornstarch into the palm of your hand. Blot over the antiperspirant using a brush or pad. Cornstarch is an extremely absorbent powder and will help you further.

Dear Diane:
I have dark spots on my legs because of bruises. I put a strong bleaching cream on them, but the spots got darker. What can I do to lighten these spots?

—Renette

Dear Renette:
Use vitamin K. Purchase the liquid or open a capsule and tap it onto the bruised areas. Vitamin K is used by surgeons to diminish scarring after surgery (especially the cosmetic type) and to treat spider veins.

Dear Diane:
I love the look I achieve with black mascara, but even waterproof brands smudge below my eyes and leave me looking like a raccoon! Do you know of any trick that won't leave me looking like one of Bambi's forest friends?

—Mary

Dear Mary:
Apply powder under your eyes *before* using your mascara. Then you can easily wipe off any flecks. Hold a tissue under your lower lash as a safeguard.

185

Dear Diane:

For years, I believed that an elegant woman should match her purse color with her shoe color. I hear the new trend is to have the purse match other accessories, like a belt or necklace, and wear shoes of a totally different color. Which is correct?

—Color Confused

Dear Color Confused:

Purse etiquette has become less hard and fast. The latest trend is to wear one color head to toe, and wear a color-contrasting purse. For instance, you could create a look by wearing black head to toe and show off your style with a bright gold purse and gold earrings.

Dear Diane:

I have unwanted hairs around my breast. Is this a common problem?

—Kiran

Dear Kiran:

This is one of the questions that's passed on to me in an anonymous note whenever it's Q&A time during one of my speeches. Stray hairs can appear anywhere on the body. You can shave the hairs off carefully with a razor. You can pluck them with tweezers. Lastly, you can opt for a more permanent solution like electrolysis or laser procedures.

Dear Diane:

About five years ago, I noticed that approximately ten minutes after applying my lipstick, it was on my teeth. It's very embarrassing! Have you ever heard of anyone else with this problem? Do you have any suggestions for me?

—Sally

Dear Sally:

This is both common and preventable. After applying your lipstick, blot your lips with a tissue. Then take that tissue and wrap it around your index finger. With your lips puckered, stick the covered finger into your mouth. Slowly draw that finger back out of your mouth, taking the excess lipstick that would have landed on your teeth on the tissue.

Dear Diane:

The skin area between my nose and lips is beginning to wrinkle. It looks like big bars, which is so unattractive. How can I remedy this?

—Brenda

Dear Brenda:

These lines can be the result of smoking or plain old genetics. You sometimes hear them referred to as "smoker's lines." The quickest way to make the lines less noticeable is to go to a health food store and get the powdered form of vitamin C. Put a small amount in the palm of your hand and add enough moisturizer to make a paste. Gently rub this mixture into the lines and leave on for thirty seconds to a minute. Then rinse. Follow up by applying the contents of a vitamin A capsule.

Dear Diane:

There are all those pills and herbs out there to "naturally" enhance breast size. Is there anything out there that might *reduce* bust size? I have the hardest time finding bras, bathing suits, and shirts that fit. Would exercise help to burn fat?

—Michelle

Dear Michelle:

Unfortunately, there is no pill or herb. Losing weight might help, but my most realistic tip is that you check out the newest minimizing bras. The latest technology reduces the appearance of the cup by a full size. Check your local department store and the major brands.

Dear Diane:

I have been trying to find the perfect close shave for a while now. Do you have any great tips? I watch the actors on TV and they have really close shaves. Is it just makeup?

—Chazi

Dear Chazi,

Although shaving is never any fun, taking a little extra time does make a big difference in a smoother look and feel. Don't shave right after getting out of bed. Your skin is puffier in the morning, making stubble less visible. Another industry secret is to use hair conditioner instead of shaving cream or soap (both tend to clog the razor). And lastly, use a loofah before shaving to help shed the top layer of dead skin, removing oil and perspiration for a closer shave.

Dear Diane:

How can I keep my lipstick from spreading into the tiny cracks around my lips? I use a lip liner pencil, but it still doesn't work. I've also tried coating my lips with pressed powder first and a store bought preparation (a gel) that is supposed to help. Nothing works. What is the secret?

—Pat

Dear Pat:

Let's get your lips pouty perfect right away! The first step is to coat your lips, not with pressed powder but with a lip conditioner like petroleum jelly or bag balm. Then, gently brush your lips to remove any flaking or chapping. Now, open your mouth wide and apply a neutral-colored lip liner. This is key to a perfect application. Finally, use a lip brush to apply your lipstick. Blot and then stick a tissue-covered finger into your mouth and pull out any excess lip color.

Dear Diane:

I have heard that as we get older, using eyeliner under the eyes is a makeup no-no. Is this true?

—Julie

Dear Julie,

Don't believe those rules that they try to make for those of us who are a certain age. A smoky eye is one of the most attractive ways to both disguise lines and give the eye definition. Use a soft eye pencil and rim around the entire eye. Then soften the look with a matching powdered eye shadow. The secret is to smudge slightly.

Dear Diane:

I accidentally picked up a permanent bottle of dye at the store and colored my hair a horrible shade of red. Is there any fast way to fade the color or to fix my hair?

—Danielle

Dear Danielle:

There are two ways you can fade out the excess color. A regular dandruff shampoo will gradually strip away the color, or you can use a mild dishwashing detergent. I prefer the dandruff shampoo because it will not jeopardize the hair shaft. Good luck! And remember to lather, rinse, and repeat!

Dear Diane:

I never had problems with a double chin before I turned 55. Are there any tricks you can give us older women to obscure this defect a little, especially when we're in the summer sunlight? Would tanning help?

—Nancy

Dear Nancy,

Although I don't ever recommend tanning, I would suggest a little self-tanner under the jaw line, followed by some light bronzing powder. It's a trick I often use to slim down the face.

189

Another suggestion is to use a slightly darker foundation under the jaw line. Always be sure to blend thoroughly.

Dear Diane:
I have naturally dark brown hair, which I dyed a lighter brown some time ago. Now the dye is slowly growing out and I don't want to renew it. However, I don't like the dye line either. Is there a natural remedy I can use to hasten this process along?

—Peta

Dear Peta:
You'll love this natural treatment. Not only does it create temporary color until your original color returns, but it also provides a lovely shine. Combine a half-cup vinegar with a quarter-cup soy sauce. Leave it on for about twenty minutes on unwashed hair, then shampoo thoroughly.

Dear Diane:
I have pale, ruddy skin and blue circles under my eyes. I don't wear makeup—I just use cover stick to try to hide those nasty things that make me look tired all the time. As I'm getting older (I'm over forty), it's been harder to hide them. I even dust the area after the cover stick has been applied and those darn circles are still there. How can I hide them but still look natural?

—Celeste

Dear Celeste,
I hope this tip helps you and your eyes: add a little yellow eye shadow to your concealer to color-correct the blue undertones.

# Chapter 17

# SITES, RESOURCES, AND FREEBIES

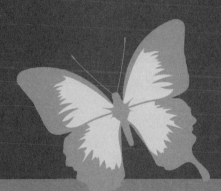

Here are some sites and hotlines that you can use. Some are commercial, but contain tips and other information along with their selection of products.

# AGING & HEALTH

www.menopause.org

www.womenssexualthealth.com

www.surgimenopause.com

www.healthboards.com

www.womens-wellness.com

www.mamassecrets.com

www.globalaging.org

www.womenco.com

www.nih.gov

## BREAST CANCER SUPPORT

Y-ME will connect you with a breast cancer survivor and provide information on support groups in your area. They will also support you in starting your own group.

800-221-2141

## GENERAL CANCER SUPPORT

800-4-CANCER (226237)

# BEAUTY SITES

www.Beauty care.com

www.beauty scene.com

www.beautyofasite.com

# DIET & FITNESS

www.ediets.com

www.womenboard.com

www.womensupportingwomen.com

www.mayoclinic.com

## AMERICAN DIETETIC ASSOCIATION

800-366-1655

# FASHION & SHOPPING ADVICE

www.fashionmall.com

www.focusonstyle.com

http://thetrendreport.com

www.saleshound.com

www.buyitonline.com

# FREEBIES

www.all-free-samples.com

www.freebiejunkie.com

http://allfreebeautysamples.com

www.free-makeup-samples.com

www.bestdealsontheweb.net

www.thefrugalshopper.com

www.freemania.net

www.gogoshopper.com

www.beautyproductssearch.com

www.freestuffkingdom.com

www.freestuffsearch.com

www.fatcatcafe.com

www.2000freebies.com

www.weeklyfreebie.com

www.freestuffshare.com

www.coolfreebielinks.com

www.freechannel.net

www.top20free.com

www.freebieville.com

# GENERAL ISSUES

www.widemedia.com

www.ivillage.com

www.ourbodiesourselves.org

www.thirdage.com

# HAIR

www.robertcraig.com
www.salonweb.com
www.hairboutique.com
www.hairdos.com
www.afrohair.com
www.hair-news.com
www.nappyhair.com
www.clairol.com
www.hairtoday.com

# SKIN CARE

www.dermadoctor.com
www.dermatologistrx.com

# PRODUCT REVIEWS

www.epinions.com
www.bizrate.com

# Final Words

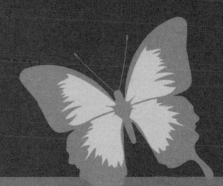

There is an age-defying movement going on, and we are all part of it. Most days we will not feel our age. How old we feel and how old we look will continually be at odds. I hope that I've been able to provide you with a few ways to make the two come together and coexist.

Age-defying methods are like spokes on a wheel. There are many ways to get there, whether you choose to do it surgically or naturally. It's your life and your body, and the way you choose to age is your choice. Just age well, and be well.

I'm reminded of Satchel Paige, the legendary baseball pitcher. He didn't even make it to the major leagues until he was in his forties. When asked about his incredible stamina, he replied, "How old would you be if you didn't know how old you was?"

Stay ageless forever.

# Index

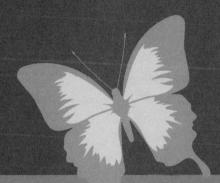

# A

# B

# ABOUT THE AUTHOR

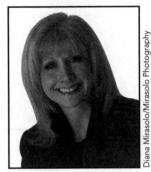

Diane Irons began her modeling career at the age of fourteen and then moved on to become a highly successful journalist and internationally known fashion and image expert.

Her investigative reporter's approach to beauty, diet, and the cosmetics industry has helped thousands of women realize that glamour and style are within their reach.

Her life's mission continues to be to bring out women's inner and outer beauty, no matter what their age, size, or budget.

Diane lives near Boston.

For more information on Diane, visit her website at www.dianeirons.com.